Yoga Psychology

Yoga Psychology

✦

The Science of the Inward Connection

Robert C. Leslie

iUniverse, Inc.
New York Lincoln Shanghai

Yoga Psychology
The Science of the Inward Connection

iUniverse books may be ordered through booksellers or by contacting:

iUniverse
2021 Pine Lake Road, Suite 100
Lincoln, NE 68512
www.iuniverse.com
1-800-Authors (1-800-288-4677)

ISBN-13: 978-0-595-39368-8 (pbk)
ISBN-13: 978-0-595-83764-9 (ebk)
ISBN-10: 0-595-39368-3 (pbk)
ISBN-10: 0-595-83764-6 (ebk)

Printed in the United States of America

Contents

Preface

In 1987 I left a position teaching psychology at a branch of the State University of New York in order to retrain as a psychological counselor and to teach yoga. I had been a student of *raja yoga* since 1959, and, having received my teacher's permission to teach on my own, taught a one-credit course in yoga meditation in addition to my traditional academic psychology courses. Over the years it became apparent that teaching yoga was more personally rewarding than lecturing to large classes of undergraduates.

I moved with my family to California where I assumed I would find plenty of people eager to study yoga. It did not take long to realize my error. The yoga that I had studied for many years emphasized the practice of concentration in a spiritual quest for self-knowledge. Such a quest required students to look deeply within and face their fears in order to let them go. This meant letting go of habitual defensiveness and cherished personal preferences.

What I found in California was that while many claimed an interest in yoga and other paths, the last thing they wanted was to face their inner demons. They preferred to cling to their habitual preferences and desires. Their interest was primarily in physical fitness and "looking good" or in finding ways to decorate their egos with magical and mystical experiences.

What they and many others fail to realize is that traditional yoga has *always* been about recognizing and knowing your innermost Self. This psycho-spiritual aim was made clear in the *Upanishads* a millennium before the time of the Buddha who himself lived 500 years before Christ.

Please understand that I am not saying there is no interest in genuine spirituality in the West. Clearly there is. The growth of Buddhist, Hindu and similar groups in the West gives evidence of a spiritual hunger not satisfied by conventional Judeo-Christian religions. Many Buddhists, however, fail to appreciate the yogic roots of Buddha's own teaching and accept the popular view that yoga is nothing but physical exercise. As for the Hindu groups they tend to emphasize a devotional or otherworldly mystical approach that departs in significant ways from the classical yogic tradition.

I write, therefore, to present yoga as a non-religious, non-mystical, *psycho-spiritual* discipline in which physical training may be a part, but remains secondary to the inward work of recognizing one's True Self-nature. I call this discipline yoga *psychology* to distinguish it from systems devoted only to physical fitness.

What I present is an understanding based on my personal practice under the mentorship of a teacher. It is not a product of academic scholarship. You may find the odd reference now and then, but what you read is largely what I have found out through practice.

Do not conclude from this that I make any claims of mastership or other forms of achievement. I assure you that I am an ordinary human being, no one special. If you read on you will, I hope, discover that traditional yoga has nothing to do with either material or spiritual attainments. It has only to do with letting go of misery.

Yoga psychology is primarily founded upon the teachings to be found in the *Yogasutra of Patanjali*. That work is a collection of 195 aphorisms written down around 200 C.E. These aphorisms provide the bare bones of a system of psycho-spiritual training. It is assumed that the serious student will find a teacher to guide the aspirant in putting flesh on those bones.

Practice is defined in yoga as any effort aimed at steadying your mental process. This is usually done through concentrative meditation, i.e., concentration on a single thought, image, sound, etc. This effort is not intellectual, but internal and experiential.

Such practice does not require that you accept any creed or dogma. Instead you are encouraged to work on yourself to bring about an awakening to your own inward Truth beyond the reach of words and concepts. You are expected to test the teachings for yourself and not accept them simply because others say you should. Similarly, there is no appeal to salvation through magic, esoteric knowledge, or divine intervention. Real yoga is not religion as will be explained later.

You should know that when you take up yoga psychology you embark on a path of ruthless self-investigation. The point is to dispel the web of ignorance and social hypnosis that keeps you from recognizing your True Self-nature. Yoga psychology intends that you find *your own* answer to the question, "Who am I?" Never let others define you.

Do not think that a search for your True Self-nature is just another egocentric self-indulgence. Your True Self-nature is not your ego or any other facet of your individual and very ephemeral personality. Your True Self-nature is your *true identity beyond birth and death*. It is what Zen Buddhists refer to as your "original face".

Do not, however, conceive of the recognition of your True Self-nature in mystical, occult, or even transpersonal terms. Yoga psychology does not promise transport to otherworldly realms or supernatural experiences. There is no unlocking of secret codes framed by Himalayan masters or Renaissance magicians. There is no promise of *personality* "transformation", "integration", or "transcendence". It is best to forget about such things. The work of yoga psychology is entirely about dismantling the machinery of misery in the here and now of your immediately lived world.

Practice is always best done under the guidance of a qualified teacher. What does it mean to be "qualified"? It has nothing to do with licenses or certificates. It does mean that a teacher has faced enough of his/her own inner demons so that s/he can support you in facing yours.

A teacher must be able to hold up a mirror to you so that you will be brought face to face with yourself. How else can you learn what you need to let go? Facing yourself is the first step to letting go of the lies and delusions that cause misery. To be a student of yoga psychology you cannot shy away from this challenge. Know also that a real teacher will not let a need for income or admiration interfere with this task.

My own teacher provided an unrelenting mirror to his students so that we might recognize what must be let go and proceed "naked" into the world. Whenever he found one of us leaning on something unnecessarily he would point it out. If that person did not let go of it he would knock it out from under them. He never did this, however, without first ensuring that the student had found sufficient inward strength to stand without such crutches. That was a mark of true compassion.

It has been my good fortune not only to find a real teacher, but also to have fellow students as models of how to apply his teachings in daily life. These fine people are constant reminders to me that in this era of blatant materialism you can practice true yoga while remaining active in the world. Putting self-discipline to work in all manner of situations they apply themselves to realizing their inherent freedom from misery.

I have also been blessed with a wife and family who allow me to indulge my practice and the sometimes "strange habits" it involves. Juggling the practice of yoga with family life is not an easy task. Some would say it is impossible. I like to think that it forced me to realizations that I otherwise would never have had.

In this modern era more and more people find themselves addicted to alcohol, drugs, food, sex, power, thrills, etc. It has been said that underlying these addictions is a craving for spiritual fulfillment, a drive to feel connected with a reality greater than the mundane and merely personal. These addicts are legion for they include us all in one way or another. They search for this connection by clinging to the outer world of mundane experience. It is my hope that this book might lead some to seek that connection within.

1

Introduction: Reality, Self, and the Ephemeral World.

Yoga psychology describes a pathway to freedom from misery. Misery (e.g., fear, anxiety, insecurity, worry, frustration, aggravation, embarrassment, etc.) arises from Ignorance of your True Self-nature. Due to this Ignorance you seek security in all the wrong places, identify with a false view of your self, and end up living a life of delusion. Under the influence of delusion your mind is like a computer infected with a virus at its deepest levels. Such a mind constructs only misery.

To wipe your mind clean of this delusion you need to re-educate yourself. You must learn to let go of Ignorance and recognize your True Self-nature. Then, free of delusion, your mind will radiate Joy without your having to seek it.

What is your True Self-nature? Have you ever looked within and asked, "Who am I?" This is *the* fundamental question and no one other than you can possibly answer it. You must also know that a real answer can be neither conceptual nor the product of some social convention. A true answer must arise from within you and be a *lived* answer. In other words, the question, "Who are you?" does not ask for words and ideas, but for you to *be* yourself.

To be yourself you must first find yourself. That is never easy for the deluded. Believe me when I say that your "True Self-nature", while it is inherently self-evident, is normally shrouded by Ignorance. Finding yourself usually means chopping your way through a jungle of lies and misconceptions. This takes work.

Before describing this work, let me indulge in a little philosophy. Yoga psychology is not philosophy, but the conceptual exercise can help to set the stage if you don't take it too seriously. According to modern yoga psychology, your True Self-nature is beyond words, but if you must say something about it you may call it "Absolute Being", "Pure Being", or simply, "Being". These words are intended to denote a reality that is permanent and not ephemeral. Simply put, Being is not subject to change.

Being manifests in many ways, e.g., *being this* and *being that*. For example, when I ask, "Who are you?" you most likely answer by saying something like, "I am female (or male), 35 years old, a teacher, live in New York City, and am a citizen of the U.S.A., etc." In other words you answer, "I am" followed by this or that detail of your personal history and life. Such statements focus attention on the "this" and "that". The "I am" tends to fade out of focus. The "I am", however, is what points to Being.

The particulars of your personal life and history, the "this" and "that", are all drawn from your sensory-perceptual and cognitive experience. Yoga psychology teaches that this realm of personal experience and cognition is entirely ephemeral and relative. That is, it involves things that are not permanent and are completely dependent on the causes and conditions of the material world. Yoga psychology further teaches that if you are to realize your inherent freedom from misery you need to shift your focus away from these ephemera to the "I am".

Why is this so? When you are feeling insecure you naturally want to grab and hold onto something solid and dependable. Yoga psychology teaches that there is nothing solid and dependable in the world of sensation, perception, and cognition. It is all subject to change. There is nothing in nature and experience that has permanence. There is nothing you can depend upon that will not, at some time or another, prove to be temporal and insubstantial. Another way of saying it is that all things in nature are born, grow old, and die.

Please understand that this is not the same as saying that the realm of nature and experience is illusory. Nature is not an illusion. If all experiences were illusions you could never reach out and *actually* touch something. You could never compare your experiences of nature with others and arrive at some consensus about what is actually present. The world of nature and experience is full of *actuality* that you can touch, see, and hear. The point is not that it is illusory, but that it is not in any way *absolutely* dependable. The world of nature and experience is not a good place to search for a lasting source of security. This is one of the most important principles of yoga psychology.

It is also important to have some sense of the relationship between the relative world of nature and experience on the one hand and Being on the other. This relationship can be difficult to conceptualize without getting lost in metaphysical jungles and I do not wish to drag you into metaphysics. The Buddha, a great teacher of yoga psychology, taught that metaphysical discussions do not lead to enlightenment. Nonetheless it may be useful to you to have some way of viewing the relationship between nature and Being. I offer two views that I have found useful (as opposed to absolutely satisfying).

I like to think of Being as the *ground* of all experience in the same way that a sheet of paper provides a ground for the words written on it. The paper makes the appearance of writing possible, and in like manner Being, as ground, makes all appearances (i.e., experiences, phenomena) possible.[1]

The other image involves the sea with its many swells, waves, and currents. Essentially, the sea is seawater and nothing but seawater, whatever form it takes. When the surface of the sea is *absolutely calm* its ultimate nature, as pure seawater, is self-evident. When the surface of the sea becomes disturbed, however, attention is captured by the individual waveforms, and their true nature as seawater overlooked, forgotten. Then it becomes easy to get lost in the details.

These details, of course, represent the ephemeral forms of nature and experience and the sea is the Great Ocean of Being. The forms of nature and experience emerge from the ground of Being in the same way that the waves emerge from the sea. They rise and they fall. Each individual waveform appears and then disappears, is born and dies. All the time, however, there is nothing but seawater. At any one moment each waveform, at whatever stage in its individual process of emergence, is *simultaneously* a transient form *and* pure formless seawater.

Similarly, your individual personhood is a process of the ephemeral realm of nature and experience. It is temporary and relative. Your individual existence is always in relation to a milieu of other individual existences, the animate and inanimate environment. That personal existence emerged from that milieu and will one day "remerge" with it. It was born and it will die.

Do not forget, however, that while your individual personhood is ephemeral it is an emergent of the Great Sea of Being. Its process is indivisible from the Greater Process of Being. From its beginning to its end, your individuality is a manifestation of Pure Being and a participant in its process of *infinite generativity.*

You might think of yourself as having a dual existence with two complementary identities. One identity involves your individual body and the socially constructed personality you have learned to associate with it. That identity is temporary; it was born and it will someday die. The other identity is your Being, the ground from which your bodily existence emerges. This latter identity is the "I am" as opposed to the "I am this and that".

To identify only with your bodily personhood is to identify with what is ephemeral and that identification leads to misery. It is wise, therefore, to educate

---

1.   The concept of Being as the ground of experience is from John Welwood. Meditation and the Unconscious: A New Perspective. In John Welwood (Ed.) *The Meeting of the Ways*, New York: Schocken (1979).

yourself to "see through" your bodily individuality and recognize your Being. *It may be even wiser to see through all such conceptualization as nothing but "mind fog" and learn to face "what is".*

None of this may be easy to accept if it goes against your cultural conditioning. Most of that conditioning took place before you had any ability to exercise critical reflection. It was as if you had been handed a script written by others and then hypnotized (socialized is the polite term) into identifying with your assigned role. Yoga psychology asserts that you can de-hypnotize yourself to unlearn that role and rewrite your script. Furthermore, you can do it in a way that keeps you from getting stuck in just another role. This is because when you recognize your True Self-nature you have a base from which to join the process of infinite generativity and create whatever role best suits your current situation.

You might look at it this way: you didn't ask to be born and you most likely didn't sign up for personal death either. In between these two "events", however, lies your individual ephemeral life. It is the "playing field" on which you learn to operate your bodily vehicle. As you stand on that playing field *karma*, the universal law of cause and effect, will compel you to act. As a creature of nature you cannot avoid the workings of *karma*. You thus have two choices. One is to let existing habits, causes, and conditions dominate how you play. In that case you may doom yourself to a feeble repetition of your past. Your other choice is to practice discipline and acquire the skills and courage to lead a truly creative life.

The latter choice, the way of yoga psychology, requires courage and a willingness to face your self. In the interests of comfort and false security, few choose it. It is a hard way that calls for *practice* rather than the consolations of philosophy, and the cultivation of *desirelessness* rather than the accumulation of either material or spiritual attainments. Yoga psychology teaches, however, that it is the only choice that leads away from misery toward Joy.

Practice in yoga psychology is any effort to steady or quiet your mind. Only a truly quiet mind offers the clarity that allows you to see through delusion and recognize Truth. The yoga tradition teaches that when your mind is infected by Ignorance, its processes will produce only misery. Practice is aimed, therefore, at quieting your mind so that Ignorance can be rooted out and your True Self-nature recognized.

I said that this way of yoga psychology is hard and few choose it. While there may be many who pursue the outer trappings not many are able to engage the inward discipline. Know then that should you embark on the path of yoga psychology you will find no crowd. The crowd seeks the easy way and you will have chosen the hard. You will encounter others, but much time will be spent alone.

You will need to learn to build *security within* rather than seek it through conformity.

This does not mean that you can look down your nose at others from on high. There is nothing to be gained from such an attitude. Such comparisons are an egocentric game of ignorance. When you choose the path of yoga psychology you choose a path that has no better and worse, no high and low. Forget about others in that regard and learn to work on your self.

Is this self-centered? What about compassion and helping others? Let me ask you, can the blind lead the blind? When you can see the Truth yourself then you *may* be in a position to show someone else the way. Until that time the best course is to work on yourself; i.e., practice inward silence, let go of your opinions, and cultivate non-attachment and a clear presence of mind. Then perhaps your actions will be spontaneously helpful to others without your even knowing it!

Yoga psychology is a discipline that requires the development of discernment, self-examination, and the courage to go one way while the crowd goes another. It requires that you learn to see through your delusions and let go of them. Delusions are like empty suitcases that you can better travel without. If you study the crowd you will see that most carry quite a bit of baggage. Learn to put your baggage down and go naked into the world.

One delusion you must overcome is that you are a separate ego, a distinct individual identified with a body. This issue will come up again and again in this work, but know now that when yoga psychology asks you to look within yourself for Truth it is not encouraging egocentrism. On the contrary, the inward work of yoga psychology asks you to "see through" ego and its multitude of fictions in order to discover the "roots" of your mind.

Yoga psychology is primarily an inward discipline, but it does not neglect the outward life. After all, your outer life is recognized as manifestation of Being. Thus, as a creature of ephemeral nature and a manifestation of Being you have a double duty. One is to work on yourself to recognize your True Self-nature, your True Being. Your second duty, complementary to and supportive of the first, is to realize fully whatever human potential resides in your temporary bodily individuality. This latter duty calls for dedication to personal *authenticity*. Let me tell you a story.

Once upon a time there was a tiger cub whose mother was killed by hunters. A ewe that had recently lost her lamb adopted it. The ewe, doing the very best she could, raised the tiger cub as a lamb. The tiger cub, naturally, had a terrible time. When it tried to "baa" it growled. The other sheep called it "stupid". When it tried to play games with the lambs it couldn't get the hang of gamboling, and the others complained it was too rough. The cub felt inferior, a failure.

One day the lambs and cub were down by a lake getting a drink of water. Suddenly, a huge fully-grown tiger appeared on the other side. "Run, it's old man tiger!" shouted the lambs and they all took off in a panic. The cub (thinking himself to be a lamb) also panicked and ran. In a few long leaps, however, the big tiger caught up to the cub and grabbed him by the scruff of his neck. "What on earth are you doing playing with these lambs? You're not one of them, you're a tiger like me. You should kill one of those stupid lambs and make a meal of it." The very thought of such a thing terrified and sickened the little tiger. Under "lamb hypnosis" he protested that he was not a tiger, but a lamb. The old tiger then dragged him over to the pond and made him look in the mirror of its surface. "Look in the water," he demanded, "do you look more like me or one of those fluffy lambs?" The cub was dumbfounded and didn't know what to say. While the cub stared at its image in the pond, the old tiger chased down and killed a lamb that had carelessly wandered too close. He then dragged the cub over and commanded, "Eat! You're a tiger and it is your true nature to eat this lamb." He forced the cub to take a bite and swallow. At first the tiger cub gagged on the meat, but then something strange happened. The raw meat began to taste wonderful. The cub tore at the meat and gulped it down. For the first time in his young life he began to feel truly alive. He lifted his head and roared with Joy. He had found himself.

The tale speaks to authenticity, i.e., to being true to your relative creaturely self. Living in accord with your natural potential is one way of expressing your True Self-nature since it is through your relative self that you manifest Being, the Absolute. At first the cub did not know how to express its nature. It had tiger-nature, but had been taught to think like a lamb. It tried hard to live like a lamb, and this caused it great misery. The cub remained in psychic pain until it was forced to look into the mirror and begin its re-education. Goaded to act according to its own relative nature it finally recognized its pathway to Joy.

In yoga psychology the experience of Joy is conceived to be the feeling consequence of your opening to Being. This opening occurs when you let go of defensiveness, clinging, and trying to be something that you are not. When you live an authentic life you open your ephemeral personhood to Being. The resulting experience is Joyous.

The story of the tiger cub also portrays a relationship between a teacher (the adult tiger) and a student (the cub). The cub is not initially happy with its teacher because it asks the cub to go against its socially constructed personality. Nonetheless, the teacher's forceful support and encouragement are consistent with the cub's own creaturely nature and leads it to its Truth. The teacher allowed the cub to discover its own confidence and break the hypnotic social trance that had to that time confined him in an inauthentic role.

As a dog must bark, bury bones, and chase cats in order to know Joy, and as a cat must chase mice, run from dogs, and scratch furniture in order to know Joy, you also must learn to live according to your creaturely nature. When you live an authentic life, acting according to your own relative nature and developing your innate capacities, Joy arises spontaneously within.

You, however, are a human being and not a cat or dog. Your choices are vastly more diverse by virtue not only of your physical attributes, but also your consciousness. Human awareness carries with it the potential for living way beyond the mere satisfaction of innate drives and desires and even beyond the development of talents and aptitudes. Human beings can learn to train themselves to become *fully present* to "what is" apart from a narrow attention to specific goals. To be sure, human beings can pursue goals according to their creaturely natures and know the Joy that it brings. At the same time they can learn to free themselves of the tyrannies of desire. This is tricky, but it can be done.

Yoga psychology calls your human potential your "duty nature". Understand that you do not need to know (ahead of time) exactly what your duty nature is. You *do* need to know that *action with presence of mind* will allow it to unfold. It takes action to convert your personal potential into a dynamic manifestation of Being. To be yourself truly you must attend to "what is" and act accordingly.

As you act you are informed by the consequences of those actions. If you pay attention to your actions and their consequences you will learn what works and what doesn't, i.e., what brings joy and what only adds to your miseries. When you pay attention to what you are doing you move from being a simple social robot to manifesting as *Conscious Being*.

And here is the tricky part: Do not let yourself become *attached* to the consequences of your actions. Try not to harbor concern about success and failure. To do so is to attend not to the present, but to a future that is only a fantasy. This, of course, includes letting go of worries about what others will think. Such concerns can only inhibit your actions, make them hesitant and awkward. Fear will freeze you. If you allow fear of consequences to take control you will get nowhere and learn nothing. The *spiritual* athlete trains hard, but *without attachment* to winning and losing.

Concepts of success and failure are truly irrelevant. They are not a good way to construe your situation whatever it may be. The tiger cub did not first fail and then succeed. Rather, it was lost and then found its self. There was never any competition or comparison other than in the *conditioned minds* of the lambs and the cub. Once the cub tasted Truth, thoughts of competition and comparison, success and failure, or embarrassment and frustration, gave way to Joy.

Only *you* can find yourself. Therefore, try not to worry about what others may be thinking or trying to put in your own head. They have nothing to do with you in regard to your own creaturely project. Practice indifference to their judgments. Heed the advice of the *Bhagavad Gita* when it teaches that, whatever the outcome, it is more blessed to pursue your own duty than receive rewards for pursuing someone else's. Just because your parents want you to be a doctor doesn't mean that it's your natural duty. Maybe you would be happier as a helicopter pilot or a chef!

This is equally true for others. You cannot realize someone else's Truth for them. You can offer support and avoid making judgments, but they have to do the necessary work. By all means share what has worked for you, but realize that it may not be the way for another.

It is important to understand that not all talents and abilities will be developed to their fullest, and not all goals that you set may be met. Real Joy arises from intent and focused effort, not from the attaining of goals. Yes, the gaining of a goal can be a cause of celebration, but such experiences do not last. No experience lasts. Know this and beware!

As an individual personality you cannot avoid the comings and goings, the ups and downs, of nature and experience. The individual waves of the sea of Being always rise and fall, appear and disappear. Along the way you will surely encounter adversity for that is the nature of things. Not all goals will be met or all talents fully realized. Remember, however, the advice of the sage *Kungfuzi* when he cautioned that while the birds of misfortune must fly over your head from time to time, you do not have to let them make nests in your hair.

Much of being your self is learning to make the best use of whatever circumstances arise. Consider life's circumstances to be your alchemical laboratory where you study, explore, and experiment with the materials that nature and experience provide. Try not to label them either good or ill, but see them as they are. That way you may discover that there is always an opportunity to turn base matter into gold. Isn't that preferable to letting every pain or adversity become a misery?

If you would become a student of yoga psychology and free yourself of misery you must learn to face nature and experience and work with it according to the shapes and forms of your relative self. You must also learn to "see through" the ephemera of nature and experience and recognize your True Self-nature. Do not let fear stop you. Root your self in Truth, and from that base become a relentless student of your own place in the world of nature, experience, and Being. Learn all you can about your relative biological, psychological, and socio-cultural natures. Amidst these manifestations of Being you will find the tools to cope with life's ups and downs and realize *your inherent freedom from misery*. Let us begin with the study of your own mind.

2

Matter, Mind, and Imagination.

In order to disentangle yourself from Misery you need to understand the nature of your own mind. In particular you need to learn how to "see through" its various "layers" and processes in order to realize their entirely ephemeral nature. Such realization allows you to let go of Misery.

The most direct path to this understanding is through meditative introspection. This introspection is not a rational analysis or other verbal process, but a *direct seeing* into the nature of your own mind through the cultivation of mental silence. Since no reading in this or any book can substitute for meditative inner work I suggest you waste no time in turning to Appendix A. It contains instructions for a simple meditation exercise. You may of course read on without first looking into this, but your study may remain merely intellectual.

Know first of all that *your mind is not an entity.* What you call "mind" is an ever changing constellation of processes. Some of these are usefully conceived as functions of your brain and its many bodily connections. Others are better viewed as interactions between you and your environment, the most important of these being social and linguistic.

The term "mental process" can sound a bit "stuffy" at times. I will sometimes use the word "mind" to avoid this. At other times I keep to "mental process" so that you will be reminded that your mind is not a "thing".

Yoga psychology's "story" of the emergence of your mental process is not a description of a longitudinal developmental sequence. Yoga psychology is not concerned with how mind develops from infancy through seniority. Yoga looks more closely at how mental processes *emerge continuously*, from moment to moment, in the way that waves emerge from the sea.

What is important to yoga psychology is the emergence of certain critical features of human *subjective experience* as revealed through meditative introspection. These features may be conceived either structurally or functionally. Structurally, they may be viewed as a series of "layers" or "envelopes" emanating from a central source, your True Self-nature. As they emerge they tend to obscure that source. To recognize your True Self-nature and find release from misery you must learn to "see through" these layers and realize that they are not identical with your True Self-nature.

It is also of value to appreciate how these processes *function* in the construction of your experience, i.e., in the creation of your world of nature and experience. To best understand both the structural and functional aspects of mental process it may help to return to the metaphor of the sea.

As waves emerge from the sea, nature and experience emerge from Pure Being. In this context nature and experience are construed as comprised of temporary "constellations" of processes that we can call "minds". Again, these minds are not self-contained independent entities, but processes essentially indistinguishable from the Sea of Being.

There are several other things about these "minds" that you need to know. (1) Like waveforms or white caps these minds emerge and remerge, appear and disappear. They are entirely transitory. (2) Mental functioning may be viewed as part of your *biological* nature, i.e., neuronal process. What you experience is a function of neural events. In other words, all of your nature and experience is a product of material mental process. (3) No mind stands independent of its environment. As you gaze upon individual waveforms in the sea it is difficult to know, precisely, where one begins and another ends. *Continuity* is much more characteristic of this "play" than is *individuality*. (4) For human minds, the most significant environment is other human minds. Your mind *depends* upon relationships with other minds. (5) A most significant feature of these relationships is *language*. Your temporary and relative identity (as opposed to your True Self-nature) may be conceived as a *story* or *narrative* formed by language (and associated images) through a process of social interaction.

According to Yogic tradition, your experience is "colored" by three fundamental qualities. Yoga psychology calls them *Truth, Energy,* and *Inertia.* Traditionally conceived as basic "constituents" of undifferentiated matter, it may be more helpful to think of them as fundamental *qualities* or "moods" that come and go in all aspects of nature and experience.

The *Truth* quality is marked by an experience of crystal clarity. It refers to a "clear seeing" that occurs when your mental vision is unimpaired by complications. This clarity is the ideal mental "state" for practicing yoga psychology. A clear mind exhibits an *uncomplicated calm* that permits the recognition of Truth.

The crystal clarity of an uncomplicated calm reveals the absolute Truth of your True Self-nature as well as the relative truths that are important for mastering your transient individual existence. You need to face and accept all of these in order to disentangle yourself from Misery and make your way in the world with dexterity.

The cultivation of crystal clarity (you might call it the practice of Truth) entails not only meditation but also being *honest* with yourself and others. A prerequisite for such honesty is the ability to face your own feelings. Such truth always begins at home.

The quality of *Energy* dominates your experience when you feel enthusiasm, vigor, "psyched", "high", driven, compelled, lustful, angry, etc.This experience can range from mild to very intense. At its most intense it is called mania.

Yogic tradition holds Energy to be manifest in all the *driving* forces of nature and experience. Energy is required for the appearance and growth of natural forms. Yoga psychology conceives of creation as energy at "play", and holds that the emergence of nature and experience (the world of form) is due to an ascendance of Energy breaking the initial balance of the qualities. This imbalance, with Energy dominating, produces a "will to form".

Psychologically, the will to form is the experience of desire. According to yoga psychology *all perceived forms are forms of desire.* That is, nothing comes into experience/existence unless a desire "wills" it. For example, you do not notice objects unless you have some "reason" to notice them. Without a reason (a desire) they do not "take form" in your mind.

When I was a cigarette smoker many years ago I had a habit to maintain and thus a reason to notice cigarette displays when I went to the store. I quit smoking over 40 years ago and now I seldom notice cigarettes. Usually I am not aware of them at all unless someone's smoke bothers me. Then, aversion motivates cigarettes into form once again. Also, I have feelings about the tobacco industry and health issues related to smoking. These may motivate my notice of tobacco products, etc.

The practice of yoga psychology requires Energy. You need the feeling of Energy in order to persist in practice. Yogic meditation involves concentration and that requires Energy. Energy must not be allowed to obscure Clarity, however. When your experience is *dominated* by Energy it can be difficult to perceive Truth.

This is also true of *Inertia.* Inertia refers to the qualities of darkness, opacity, solidity, heaviness, and resistance. Experiences of Inertia include sluggishness, torpor, mental dullness, and depression. Inertial feelings dominate when you lack enthusiasm and do not feel motivated to do things. Also, since Inertia involves the experience of darkness or opacity, it obscures Truth. When Inertia is dominant someone can explain something to you over and over again, but you just can't "get" it.

The three qualities, in various combinations, account for the range of moods in your experience. These begin as interior moods, but are readily *projected* onto the phenomena you perceive as the "external world". For example, you experience energy in thunderstorms and boiling liquids, etc. Inertia manifests when you feel physical mass and experience its resistance to lifting or pushing. Clarity is expressed in the feeling of clean freshness that follows a rainstorm or when you perceive some figure sharply against a background. The "aha!" of seeing the solution to a puzzle is due to Clarity coming into dominance.

Each of the three qualities is always part of your experience to some degree. Even in states of the greatest Clarity, Energy and Inertia remain "hovering in the wings". When you see an object very clearly it still involves the influence of Inertia expressed as the object's mass or solidity. Problem solving usually involves a combination of Energy and Clarity.

It is important for you to appreciate how the three qualities "flavor" your experience. Awareness of their comings and goings is part of learning how your mind works. The more you understand about the qualities the better able you are to cultivate them as needed.

Cultivating Clarity is essential to the entire practice of yoga psychology. Being able to manipulate your level of Energy is also very important. Even the quality of Inertia has its uses as in learning how to modulate Energy or become "heavy" and "immoveable" when necessary (e.g., resisting physical or social pressures).

Always keep in mind, however, that these are qualities *of experience*, i.e., qualities of the transient and ephemeral world of nature and experience. Your experience of these qualities comes and goes like any other. Therefore, it is not wise to attach yourself to any quality.

This is especially true with the quality of Truth or Clarity. By all means learn to cultivate mental Clarity, but do not cling to it. However "good" you get at your practice there will be days when things are not as clear as you want them to be. Attachment to Clarity may then bring you the misery of loss. Students of yoga psychology must avoid becoming "bliss heads" addicted to particular experiences, moods, or mental states.

The qualities are considered to be intrinsic to the "stuff" of nature and experience, i.e., "moods" of the material-mental "sea". They exist prior to the emergence of individual "minds". What now follows is an account of the emergence of minds.

Mental process begins with the emergence of *imaginative potential* or Imagination. Imagination, the creation of images, is the foundation of all experiencing and reflects a "will to form", i.e., the workings of Energy.

The formation of images is essential to the construction of all sensory and perceptual experience. Imagination, whether directly related to sensory process, evoked by words, or manifested in dreams and hallucinations, underlies all human experience as a fundamental "power" of mind. It is the root of all perception from the most mundane to the most sublime.

There are two additional processes that must be mentioned in connection with Imagination that make possible the perception of a world of forms. These are *discrimination* and *projection*.

Discrimination takes place whenever a figure is perceived against a ground as well as when one form is discerned from another. A capacity for discrimination supports the emergence of any *sensory-specific* imagery, e.g., visual images, auditory images, etc. Discrimination is essential to all sensory perceptual experience.

Discrimination is linked to the behaviors of *pointing* and (later) *naming*. When you point to a particular object you can direct someone's attention to it, i.e., you increase the chances that the object will become a perceived form for another. Naming the object helps you distinguish it from other objects, e.g., "dogs" as opposed to "cats". In most cases such names establish *classes* of objects that share certain common properties, e.g., triangles v. rectangles, or pines v. cedars. The participation of these pointing and naming functions in the ordering of your experience is why the world of nature and experience is also called "the world of *name* and form".

Projection refers to the movement outward from a source that is inherent in the process of emergence. In yoga psychology perceived forms are conceived as projected onto the "screen" of your mental movie theater. This means that what you perceive as "out there" actually originates from within your own mental process. Yoga psychology conceives of all mental emergence as arising from "within" and being projected "outwards".

If you find any of these ideas hard to swallow I suggest you keep chewing on them. They represent the experience of yogis over many millennia of inward study, and that is nothing to "sneeze" at. At the same time it is no reason to take it all on faith. You must search within and verify for yourself that what is said squares with your own experience and is useful to you. My appeal to millennia of yogic experience is made not so that you will become a parrot of yogic dogma, but that you might take the claims sufficiently seriously to do your own work and not quit at the first signs of difficulty.

3

Mental Emergence and the "I"-thought.

The powers of Imagination, especially that of *discrimination*, enable the emergence of the "I"-thought. Also called the "ego function", the "I"-thought is the beginning of self-conscious awareness.

The "I"-thought is your very first self-conscious thought and provides the ground of all subsequent self-conscious thought. Everything that goes on in your "personal mind" does so against the ground of the "I"-thought. This implies (to be verified by your own inner work) that all thought stems from the "I"-thought and can be traced back to it.

Emergence of the "I"-thought creates an *image* of your self as a *separate* being. With the "I"-thought you experience yourself as separate from "the world" and from "others". This *sense* of separation divides your perception into a seemingly observing *subject* that stands apart from a world of observed *objects*, the "world out there". Both subject and object are *products of imagination*, and their perception as separate entities depends upon the power of *discrimination*.

The apparent separation of the "I"-thought and the world is the beginning of all *dualistic* thinking. Dualistic thought structures your perception in terms of opposites or contraries, e.g., self and other, us and them, safety and danger, right and wrong, good and evil, etc. It all begins with the seeming split between a subject self and a world of objects deemed not-self.

The self-other split becomes "solidified" when the "I"-thought is identified with the body. This identification marks the beginning of Egoism and is described in more detail in Chapter IV. For now it is enough to know that the identification of the "I"-thought with the body initiates a dramatic expansion of opposites. For example, with the body as a spatial reference point, you get "near" and "far", "here" and "there", etc. As you will see in Chapter IV a most important psychological expansion of the self-other dichotomy is that into "me" and "you" and then "mine" and "yours".

By the way, do not take my word for any of this. Look within your own mind and try to see what is actually present. Study your mind and draw your own conclusions. Remember, however, that you may have to wade through layers of habit until you can see "what is".

This, by the way, is an invitation to study your self "within", and here is another dichotomy, "within" as opposed to "without". Once the body becomes a subjective point of reference the tendency is to view mental process as taking place "inside". That is, you place your "self" *inside* the body with the world of the "other" stationed "out there". Try to be aware of this as you begin to observe your own mental processes (see Appendix A for instructions on meditation).

Once the appearance of a separation between subject and object arises, the perception of subsequent mental features tends to get "sorted" along two lines, the "mental" and the "physical". This dualism is as much a cognitive construction as any other rooted in the apparent separation of subject and object. Similar dualisms that you may come across are mind-matter, spirit-matter, and subtle-gross, etc.

What you need to know is that in spite of the apparent mind-body or mental-physical dualism yoga psychology regards all "mental" and "physical" events to be part of a single *material continuum*. The only difference between mental and physical is that mental events are relatively subtle and private (or subjective) whereas physical events are relatively gross and public. Both, however, are part of the material realm of nature and experience.

The conceptualization of nature as a material continuum ranging from the very subtle to the very gross has lead to all manner of interpretive speculation. The temptation for many has been to fall into the trap of conceiving of the subtle as somehow more "spiritual" than the gross. Along with this has been a tendency to equate what yoga calls the "subtle body" with Western religious ideas about "the soul", etc. This has lead to a re-conceptualization of the material continuum of subtle-gross as a spirit-matter dualism. This is an error that will be discussed more fully in Chapter IX on tantra.

What follows is an account of the continued emergence of "mental" process. Please remember that this account is entirely conceptual. It is offered as one way of thinking about the nature of experience and how you might construct it. Only your actual practice will determine if it useful to you or not.

According to yogic tradition after the emergence of the "I"-thought and a sense of separation between subject self and object world, mental emergence splits into two directions. One path follows the emergence of those processes conceived as "mental", and thus part of the subjective order, while the other involves those conceived as "physical" and part of the object world.

The mental line of emergence (ideally dominated by the quality of clarity) includes the traditional five senses, five modes of action (the energy quality is not excluded), and cognitive organizing processes. The traditional five senses are sight, hearing, taste, touch, and smell that are largely oriented to your "external" environment or the world "out there". To these we can add senses more attuned to your "internal" environment, i.e., proprioception (skeleto-muscular sense) and interoception (sensory feedback from the activities of glands and other internal organs). The traditional modes of action include your hands, feet, speech, and excretory and reproductive organs, i.e., the means by which you act upon your world.

Meditative self-study (and much experimental research) suggests that sensory activity cannot be separated from cognitive-perceptual organization, and that both are intimately affected by your actions. What this means is that without cognitive organizing the sensory world you live in would appear chaotic and unpredictable. Nothing would "make sense" and this would cause great anxiety.

Cognitive organization is perhaps better called "cognitive construction". Its primary function is to make sense of your experience, i.e., to construct a perceived world in which you can feel "at home". This constructive process fabricates your expectations, assumptions, beliefs, and all manner of labeling and classification systems. Most important, it involves narratives.

Narratives can include a host of story styles ranging from hunting tales and creation myths to movie scripts and highly sophisticated scientific theories. The underlying motive in all cases is a search for security. Narratives attempt to describe the world and your actions in such a way as to make events predictable and/or controllable.

Another very important role of narratives is to encode social rules and structures. Myths and fairy tales for example include many images that describe what makes people "good" or "evil" and how you should behave in order to be everything from a hero, to a good ruler, parent, or simple decent person.

Since narratives begin with stories that are spoken or sung the speech function deserves special attention. Speech is the root of narrative and other forms of communication and thus has profound social and cognitive significance. The role of language in social and cognitive organization cannot be denied.

Further, much of what you call "thinking" is actually internalized speech that has its roots in social conversation. This means that linguistically mediated cognitive processes are greatly influenced by your surrounding culture via social discourse. Narratives and other forms of spoken and written discourse "store" and convey your beliefs and values.

Narratives operate at many levels of awareness. Some are so habitual that they operate automatically and unconsciously. These constitute part of the "subtle" structures that guide your perception and behavior. They operate "behind the scenes" as they structure and organize how you see your world. Usually it requires special training or circumstances to bring them into awareness.

Among these subtle organizing principles are those of space, time, and cause. For example, all perception involves some kind of spatial organization. One of the most basic aspects of this is organization in terms of figure and ground. Unless you can discern a figure apart from its background it remains virtually invisible.

When you perceive a figure against a ground your perceptual process has already organized things spatially so that the figure is salient. Generally, you do not fully notice the ground and it remains more or less "unconscious". It usually requires special coaching to get you to shift your attention to the ground. When you do, the ground or some part of it emerges as a new figure and the old figure recedes into the ground.

Art students, for example, are taught to become aware of "negative space". This refers to focusing attention on the space between figures and coming to regard it as a figure in its own right. This reveals both the interdependency of figure and ground and the role of habit in perception. It may also help you realize that space is not absolute, but relative.

Space "itself" is never an actual *object* of perception. It is a construct, a pure verbalism. We employ the word "space" to help us talk about and thus think about the world we live in. The word allows us to generalize about experiences of distance, physical separation, and place. Perhaps "space" is simply another name for "background".

If you find all of this difficult to accept do not despair. Look up "space" in a philosophical dictionary and discover how many ways it has been treated and defined. Clearly space presents a puzzle that has thus far defied consensus. But please do not take my word for it. Think about it. Meditate on it. Consider, when you look out into "space" if you actually perceive a discrete object that could bear the name?

The category of time presents a similar problem. Time is never an *object* of sensation or perception. Your "perception" of time depends entirely upon noticing *changes* that occur between two or more observations of "an object". An obvious example is the position of the sun in the sky or the movement of the hands on a clock. You notice a change of position and say that "time" has elapsed.

We have no direct experience of time so we must use metaphor to make sense of it. We frequently speak of "saving", "spending", or "running out of" time *as if* time were substance. Similarly we say that "time is money". Time, of course, is neither substantial nor is it "hard" currency. Time is entirely conceptual, a pure fancy.[1]

The metaphors allow you to *conceive* of time as both valuable and measurable. In so doing it appears to concretize time. If time were concrete it would be *present to your senses* and you would not have to employ the metaphor. The metaphor makes *sense* of time by "borrowing" the concreteness of another domain of experience.

As stated before, what you actually perceive is a change in some aspect of the material world. You then construe that change as having occurred "over time". In truth what your senses actually perceive is neither time nor change, but a sequential series of sensory images that are sufficiently similar to be construed as the same object or person, but different enough for you to decide that something must have "changed" from one to the other. For example, after having not seen an old high school classmate for some years you encounter the person and note that s/he has gained weight, now wears glasses, etc. You perceive this construction to be the "same" person you used to know, but that they have changed.

Memory is critical to such perception. Without memory you cannot make the comparisons of before and after necessary to construct change. Note also that your construction of change also depends upon the assumption that the before and after observations refer to the same person or object. Not only have you constructed change, but necessarily someone or something that undergoes change.

The conceptualization of an individual person who has continuity "across time" is interesting to consider. How do you come to the conclusion that "it" is the "same" person? I submit that you do this by weighing the similarities and differences (and this depends upon memory) such that if the similarities outweigh the differences you conclude that your observations are of the same individual. In other words, there is a threshold for determining that the differences between the images are too great to represent the same person.

Ultimately, this kind of cognitive constructing depends on the "I"-thought and projection. Initially, you collect your memories of various experiences and

---

1.   I owe these insights to G. Lakoff 's and M. Johnson 's book *Metaphors We Live By*. Chicago University Press, 1980.

knit them over your "I"-thought. That is, you begin by constructing an image of yourself as having continuity over "time". You construe memory images as "owned" by your "I"-thought and come to view the changes from day to day and year to year as "your" personal history. Without the "I"-thought you would have no "string" on which to hang your various observations. In that case you would most likely construe them as unconnected and not attached to any individual identity.

After you construct your own identity around your "I"-thought you proceed to *project* identities onto others. Since these others are busy constructing and maintaining their own identities you get no argument about identities in general and consensus reigns. Everyone is seen as having an identity, an individual personhood.

The assumption/construction of personal continuity across time and space is a powerful one that comes to dominate most of your cognitive life. Along with your assumptions about time and space it operates largely at an unconscious level and is not normally subject to scrutiny.

Another deep assumption involved in the construction of your world is that of *cause*. Normally your perception of a causal connection between events depends on your perceiving those events as having spatial and/or temporal contiguity. Your perception of causality is dependent on those constructs.

There is little question that you are much more likely to assume a causal relationship between two events if one of them reliably precedes the other "in time" and they are also "close" together in space. I believe that this constructing has been pretty much "wired in" to your brain through evolution. Much more is involved in actually *proving* that a causal relationship exists, but in your immediate experience, temporal and spatial contiguity are very compelling.

Another contribution to your assumptions about causation might include the projection of your own agency. All of us acquire some degree of experience creating objects, moving things around, and attempting other forms of "hands on" control. Since you often experience direct control of objects it is easy to assume that something or someone else controls events not under your control. Once again this is a projective assumption on your part.

The history of human belief describes all manner of spirits and occult forces that are assumed to control natural events. We do not actually sense these agents exerting control, but make the assumption nevertheless. Facing events that we do not understand we construe them in terms that we are more directly familiar with. We look about us and see all of nature in its mystery and wonder, and assume that some agent, e.g., a creator god, made it.

The "religion" of natural science offers more sophisticated explanations for natural events, but depends equally on the constructs of space, time, and cause. Whatever your belief system, from atheistic scientism through fundamentalist theism, space, time, and cause are fundamental features of your perception of the world. Without them you would not be able to construct a meaningful map of "reality" to guide you through your daily life.

These cognitive constructions thus constitute the underlying and largely unconscious structure of your developing "knowledge base". Without them you would feel lost and insecure. Consequently, testing them and keeping them up to date occupy a significant amount of your cognitive activity. This activity becomes most intense when your experience doesn't match your expectations.

Cognitive maps come in many shapes and sizes. In the natural sciences, for example, theories of varying complexity attempt to account for all manner of phenomena. Such theories guide research by organizing observations and generating testable hypotheses. When tests support a theory, researchers feel more confident and secure in their understanding of the subject matter.

When experimental outcomes don't fit the theory several things can happen. The theory may be "tweaked" to accommodate the anomalous observations. If this doesn't work, or if contrary findings become too numerous, a theory may have to be abandoned. Historically, this normally doesn't happen until a competing theory comes along that does a better job of making sense of the observations.

History also shows that theories tend to die slowly. After all they are the product of human thought and the originators can get very possessive of them. Egos get involved (and sometimes money). Theories tend to be cherished by their developers and may be defended with the tenacity of a mother bear protecting her cub.

Too often data contrary to theory are simply denied, i.e., pushed aside as if they didn't exist. No one likes to discover that the world is not the way they think it is. The failure of a theory (or any "map") to predict and explain events can cause anxiety. Like little children, therefore, we often look the other way and hope the "bogeyman" will disappear.

Human beings have a need for knowledge of their world and devote a lot of cognitive energy to constructing it and passing it on to others. This is not just something that only occupies scientists; all of us do it all the time.

A common vehicle for this is the personal story or narrative. Scientific theories may be considered stories of a sort. It is true that in science the demand for precision and rigor lessens its mass appeal. Outside of the scientific specialties most people prefer stories couched in ordinary language, i.e., a "good yarn".

Much human knowledge (e.g., information, attitudes, and beliefs) is transmitted across generations through myths conveyed as bedtime stories, folk tales, newspaper articles, or political and motivational speeches, etc. All of these usually involve some form of narrative to drive their messages home.

All good story telling is hypnotic. The gifted storyteller or rhetorician literally entrances you with a tale. Listening to a well-told story puts you in a highly suggestible state, and you are very likely to imbibe the underlying beliefs and attitudes without being aware of it. Also, when you are under the spell of a good story you are not, as a rule, able to reflect critically on its content.

The transmission of cultural knowledge through stories begins very early in life. When you consider the extreme imbalance of power that exists between adult storyteller and impressionable child you have a recipe for brainwashing. We don't like to call it brainwashing; we prefer "socialization" or "education".

First you hear stories and then you repeat them to yourself. They become part of the internal narrative by which you describe yourself and your world. These narratives often take the form of conversations between you and imagined others. They may be accompanied by images in which you engage in virtual action. The narrative and accompanying images become a running definition of you-in-the-world. The point is that you spend a good deal of your mental energy constructing and living in an imagined fictional, virtual reality.

Your narratives encompass your understanding of yourself and "what is", and thus give you a sense of meaning. To have meaning helps you feel more comfortable in the world; it salves the felt wounds of separation. The problem, however, is that neither the wound nor the salve is actual. They are imaginal. The result is a neurotic compulsion in which you believe the salve must be reapplied continuously.

This is why silence can be so discomfiting. Your narratizing could not take place without the medium of language. You learned your language and its myths at your mother's "knee" not to mention the "knees" of your father, siblings, teachers, neighbors, and peers. The language of these stories provided the "capsule" in which you "swallowed" a world-view with all its cognitive habits.

Please understand that this is so whether you swallowed the capsule easily or with difficulty. Whether you conformed to your culture gleefully or rebelled against it, the narratives shaped your existence. In this the role of internal conversation was all-important.

In your inner (and outer) narratives the "I"-thought serves as the primary protagonist and author. As the root of all thought the "I"-thought is the kernel around which the plot elements of your story are organized. Take away the "I"-thought and much of the inner narrative simply disappears.

The story elements are many, but chief among them are your *goals* and the *conflicts* that arise when you are blocked from achieving them. With the "I"-thought as the "hero" of your narrative, and your motivations and conflicts organized around it, you have the basics for virtually any plot.

The work of yoga psychology concerns itself largely with the most fundamental of human plots, i.e., the quest for security in an uncertain world. Yoga psychology studies how you and others construct knowledge maps and personal narratives in your struggles to create security in the face of a world that offers nothing but flux. Yoga psychology does this in order to know how the mind constructs misery and how that construction can be ended.

The next chapter (Chapter IV) explores the *nature of knowledge* and your attempts to use it to remove uncertainties and feel secure. Following that, Chapter V deals with the *emotional forces* that motivate your search for knowledge and security. The latter amounts to a description of the "machinery" of Misery. Then we move on to what you can do to *let go* of Misery. That, after all, is the primary aim of Yoga psychology. In this regard, if you have not already looked at the meditation instructions in the appendix now would be a good time to do so.

4

The Nature of Knowledge

Your mental process continuously engages in seeking and constructing knowledge of the world and your place in it. Without such knowledge you are like a traveler in a strange land who has neither a map nor any grasp of the local language. Your mind thus seeks knowledge in order to help you feel that you are in familiar territory and thus secure.

Unfortunately, knowledge seeking is easily subverted to the making of misery. Then your mental process creates more insecurity than it alleviates. Most people do not know how to prevent this subversion from happening and become trapped in a vicious cycle of misery. In order to prevent this, yoga psychology studies the knowledge process as a necessary prerequisite to practice.

Please understand that the generalizations presented here provide only a *conceptual* guide to the nature of knowledge. To understand your own mental process you must go beyond concepts and face yourself *within*. No one else can do that for you.

Yoga psychology's understanding of the knowledge process comes from the meditative experience of practicing yogis going back at least four thousand years. These yogis were much more interested in knowing themselves from *within* rather than knowing a world from without. They understood that genuine security could not come from knowledge of the sensory world, and therefore became empiricists of the subjective. They asked how we could ever be certain of our knowledge of a world "out there" if we did not first comprehend the nature of "the knower".

This distinction between "knower" and "known" does constitute a dualism, and you may wonder why it is used here. The dualistic conceptualization comes from *Samkhya* psychology, which was widely accepted during Patanjali's time and which he adopted. Although the dualism must be abandoned at a later point, it is much easier to use in beginning a discussion of the nature of knowledge as it conforms to common sense.

Samkhya assumes that all experience involves the interaction of a pure conscious subject or "Seer" on the one hand, and an unconscious world of material "seen" objects on the other. The Seer is called *Purusha*, variously translated as spirit, person, male, pure awareness, etc. The seen is known as *Prakriti*, a kind of great "mother nature". In the later *Vedanta* philosophy *Purusha* becomes the *Atman* or Self that is identical with *Brahman*, the absolute. Here I will use Seer or Self for *Purusha*, and Nature, or nature and experience, for *Prakriti*.

Please note that according to this view only the Seer is conscious. The world of the known, i.e., the realm of nature and experience, consists entirely of *unconscious* matter. Consciousness may penetrate matter, but always remains essentially independent of it.

Although unconscious, material nature is conceived as dynamic. Matter is thought to consist of a vast field of energy in states of constant vibration and apparent change. Matter may be unconscious, but it is full of power, the power of generativity. Without such power nature would not be able to generate the changes necessary to create experience for the enjoyment of the Seer.

What this means is that "your" knowledge and experience are not "yours". They belong only to the Seer. To think that experience and knowledge are yours is a huge egocentric error, a delusion. As you will see in the next chapter, this point is critical to an understanding of the process of yoga.

A much more critical assertion underlying yoga psychology's view of knowledge is that you cannot have any *immediate* knowledge of an external world. Your knowledge is entirely mediated by sensory, perceptual, and cognitive processes. You only experience what your mental processes present to you.

Even your experience of an external world as "out there" is dependent on your mental process's capacity to organize experience in spatial terms. This is organization from *within*. The structuring process of your mental "apparatus" imposes the categories of space, time, and cause, etc., as it shapes "your" experience. What you come to know is entirely a *construction* of your own mental process.

Does this mean that there is really no world out there? Not at all; it says that *you cannot know* what is out there, or if there really is an out there, in any *immediate* way.

Because you are limited to your own experience, only you can decide for yourself what is or is not so. This leaves you with the pragmatism of having to test your knowledge to see "what works". If actions based on your knowledge are successful you will decide that your knowledge is true. If your actions fail, however, you will doubt or reject your knowledge.

You must test your knowledge through *action* if you are ever to know what does and does not work. Only action can inform you of the validity of your maps, theories, beliefs, and other forms of knowledge.

When stimulated by sensory activity your mental process forms percepts that *represent* objects in the "world out there". The construction of these representations involves sensory processes, cognitive organization, linguistic encoding, and memory.

Although classical yoga does not emphasize it you should also be aware that your cognitive processing is influenced by your social context. You are a social being and your knowledge is influenced by what others think and believe. While your actions provide the most direct test of your knowledge you also need to consider what happens when your findings disagree with those made by others.

How do you deal with such a situation? Do you reject your own knowledge and meekly recant? Perhaps you become a rebel and defy convention. There are many ways of dealing with knowledge conflicts including learning to live with differences of opinion. The latter is made easier if you do not *cling* to your own opinions and hold them sacrosanct. In any case, do not fail to consider the effects of social influence on the formation of your knowledge.

Yoga psychology describes five classes of knowledge: right knowledge, wrong knowledge, fancy, sleep, and memory. Let's begin with the distinction between right and wrong knowledge.

Both right and wrong knowledge involve the interpretation of a perceived object. In the case of right knowledge the interpretation is valid, i.e., it conforms to the "true nature" of the object. Wrong knowledge is formed when the interpretation is faulty. For example, assume there is rope on the ground in front of you. If you perceive the object to be a rope your knowledge is right knowledge. If, however, you perceive the object to be a snake, your knowledge is wrong.

How do you know that your percept does or does not conform to "reality"? Ultimately you must test your knowledge through some action. You act on the knowledge and come to a conclusion that it works for you or does not work for you. For example, you may pick up the rope and obtain further sensory information that is consistent with your original percept. It doesn't wriggle and try to bite you so it is probably not a snake, etc.

Right and wrong knowledge may also arise from testimony. With testimony you form an image based on a report of someone else's sensory-perceptual experience. If that person's knowledge is right and their reporting is clear and accurate your mental image will be right knowledge. If the source of the testimony was mistaken or failed to provide a clear account you may construct wrong knowledge.

A third source of knowledge is inference. You may arrive at knowledge of an object by inductive or deductive reasoning. Whether or not inference leads to right knowledge will depend upon the quality of your initial observations (in the case of inductive reasoning), your premises (in the case of deductive reasoning), and the correctness of your logic in reaching a conclusion. For example, in the rope and snake case you might initially mistake a rope for a snake, but then recall that you are in Hawaii where there are no snakes and by inference conclude that your first interpretation was wrong. Or you might, if you were in Maine during January, notice that the temperature was below zero and infer that no self-respecting cold-blooded creature would be out and about.

In all cases actual testing of the knowledge is critical to see if your observations, testimony, or reasoning lead to knowledge that actually works for you. This does not mean that you must engage in the constant conscious testing of your knowledge. If you are a reasonably active person your day-to-day activities will constitute a running test of your perception, conclusions, assumptions, etc. If things work out your knowledge is serving you well. When trouble happens you know that you need to do some checking.

When some aspect of your knowledge is wrong you should eventually find out through some undesired consequence of its use. Of course if you are an agoraphobic shut-in you may never venture forth to put your knowledge to work and remain forever a prisoner of your fears and inadequate learning.

The third class of knowledge is called "fancy". Fancy refers to mental images that are not triggered by sensory activity, but by words and feelings. They include conceptualizations, daydreams, dreams, and hallucinations. The student of yoga psychology needs to understand these forms of fancy in order to become familiar with their uses and limitations.

By far the most important form of fancy is conceptualization. This is because it comprises the greatest share of your waking thought process. Conceptualizations are triggered by words, and are usually the names of *generalizations* or *classes* of objects. In other words, concept names do not denote particular objects, but rather *classes* of objects having common properties, e.g., "triangles" have the common property of three sides. The mental images evoked by such words are *concepts*.

Consider the word "pen". When you read or hear "pen" you form a sensory (visual and/or tactile) image of a pen. The image, in this case, is not evoked by an object in contact with your senses, but by the spoken or written word "pen". The word "pen" in such a case does not designate any particular pen, but the class of all possible pens. If we both hear the word "pen" you might image one kind of pen while I might image a very different one. If a speaker wanted to narrow the class s/he could say, "ball point pen" or "quill pen". The added adjectives refer to *sub classes* of pens and narrow the scope of your conceptualization. If the person had said something like, "the red pen next to your glass" while pointing to an actual pen available to your senses, the remark would refer to a specific object and not a concept.

The conceptualization of classes and sub classes is one of the ways in which you organize your mental world. Class names and labels enable you to categorize and organize your experiences of the world. Classifications superimpose a conceptual order on your experiences. This mental "housekeeping" gives you a sense of control. Everything has its "pigeon hole" and chaos is seemingly reduced. You feel more secure.

By the way, conceptualization involves your "powers" of discrimination. Any time you name and denote a class of objects you discriminate or differentiate that class from other classes of objects.

When you name an object or a person you usually increase your potential control. If you say something like, "Suzy, please hand me the pen," you are using two names to gain a specific objective. The name "Suzy" allows some control over the person named and that control is directed by the word "pen". The kind of control enabled by naming is reflected in the slang for name, "handle". It implies direct "hands on" control.

Concepts, however, cannot be handled in the same concrete way that you handle actual objects. Rather, concepts are "entertained" by your mental process and evoke images as the concept names are spoken either out loud or silently as part of an internal private discourse. This internal speaking and resulting imagery permits *virtual* manipulation of objects in your mental space.

Not all names denote classes of objects that refer back to something that can be actually handled. You also use words to name actions, relationships, and processes. Processes include practically all events in nature, the weather, seasonal cycles of growth and decay, animal and human social interactions, neurophysiological functioning, artistic production, imagining, etc.

It is misleading to think of these processes as if they were discrete objects simply because you give them names. Not all nouns denote objects you actually get your hands on, i.e., grasp. Nonetheless, the ability to name and then play with words and the images evoked gives us a kind of "grasp". This may be virtual rather than actual, but it adds to our feeling of security.

The virtual world made possible through conceptualization is very important. It enables you to construct an *imaginal* world in which you may carry out complex manipulations and interactions in virtual space. This can be imagined physical space or it can be social space. You can rotate objects, rehearse actions and conversations, make plans, or indulge in sexual fantasies.

In your virtual space you can try things out without fear of actual consequences. This expands your ability to invent and create. Artists often visualize their work before putting brush to canvas or chisel to stone. Entrepreneurs and developers imagine shopping centers, restaurants, industrial parks, and residential communities where none presently exist. Their opponents visualize air and water pollution, traffic congestion, natural habitats spoiled, and other environmental disasters. Yes, conceptualization can embody and extend all manner of conflicts.

Ultimately, however, the fruition of any imaginal process depends upon taking *action* in the *actual* world. Without action dreams remain dreams. Action is required to move you out of the virtual and into the actual. Only in the actual world can you know if your plans *actually* work or if your dreams can be *actualized*.

Of course, fear of consequences may keep you from action. In some cases you might delude yourself into thinking that virtual reality is truly safe and comfortable in the long term. Given a craving for security, the apparent safety of virtual reality can have a tempting, even addicting, allure.

To try to realize your dreams through concrete action is one thing; to remain suspended in fancy is quite another. Fancy may appear safe, but its misuse invites stagnation. By all means employ your imaginal abilities to poetize, plot and plan, but do not forget to act.

You would do well to think of concepts as dead things. Think of them as photos in an album. You may use them to stimulate imaginal activities and memories, but they are not actuality. You can look at photos and even talk to them, but they will not respond. Embracing a photo is not the same as hugging an actual loved one. Concepts are frozen and lifeless. Attachment to conceptualization leads to a life among the dead.

The construction of your virtual world depends upon memory as much as it does on conceptualization. According to yoga psychology the most important feature of memory is its *holding* onto the past. Memory allows you to keep the past in virtual space where, in league with conceptualization, it exerts influence on your present.

Yoga psychology is not particularly concerned with brain mechanisms of recollection and recall or their measurement. It focuses instead on how you might allow memory's holding to lead you to keep repeating past errors and thereby cast a gloom over your present. Memory is a vehicle of *karma* and helps tie you to the wheel of birth, death, and rebirth.

It is rebirth when you repeat mistakes over and over again or block creativity by clinging to old views and opinions. It is memory that allows you to hold onto conceptualizations of yourself that have lost their usefulness. For this reason, and others mentioned below, Yoga psychology calls memory a "binding gloom".

Memory allows you to construct a personal narrative and give yourself continuity within it. You cannot have a narrative without its "hero" and a "time line" running from the hero's past through the present and on into the hero's future. You cannot conceive of either a past or a future, and thus of yourself as a historical entity, without memory.

Memory reconstructs images of your interactions with others, providing a social context. This context includes your attitudes and beliefs, those of significant others, and importantly, how those others may have regarded you. These memories are, to a greater or lesser extent, "owned" by you as part of your egocentric complex and become part of how you see yourself in the world. In other words, the narratives that others tell about you become grafted into your own personal narrative in one way or another.

Your personal narrative is constructed from processes of memory and conceptualization. In the present it normally takes the shape of a running internal dialogue centered on "I"-thought as narrative "hero". Put this against the background of a recollected past and projected future and you have the essentials of your personal identity.

This is not the end of the construction of your personhood, and we must come back to it in the next chapter. For now it is enough to understand that your personal narrative and identity are, essentially, *constructions* of fancy and memory.

We come at last to dreams, daydreams, and hallucinations. Modern yoga psychology classifies these as fancy because they are not immediately evoked by sensory stimulation. They are perceptual-cognitive productions generated by cognitive-emotional needs.

Although dreams occur during your sleep, and hallucinations occur when you are awake, the imaginal processes involved are essentially the same. You may think of hallucinations as waking dreams.

Generally, dreams and hallucinations express feelings and emotions that you are unable to express consciously because to do so would generate intolerable anxiety. Such anxiety arises because the feelings are inconsistent with your preferred images of self and/or the world, e.g., images of being safe, loved, strong, a nice person, capable, etc.

Dream imagery usually represents experiences that you have never properly assimilated to your cognitive schemas. This means that you have bits and pieces of experience that do not fit your normal way of looking at things. As a result you cannot "swallow" them and they stick in your psychic craw resulting in a state of cognitive-emotional imbalance.

Your cognitive process constructs dream images as an attempt to restore psychic balance. Your dream process will continue to construct images until the "loose ends" are knitted into a coherent and manageable structure and balance restored.

Since this process usually represents a challenge to your established schema it can cause considerable discomfort. This is why most dreams are at least mildly disturbing and often quite terrifying.

Dreams express their content in a way that ignores the strictures of everyday waking language. Dreams do not observe the "niceties" that you employ to avoid ruffling the feathers of other people. Dreams follow emotional expression rather than logic and are largely composed of non-verbal sensory images that tend to defy socially consensual ways of constructing experience. It is no wonder that your dreams often appear weird.

The language of dreams is a kind of body language. I do not refer to postural signals, but to a non-verbal vocabulary of bodily activities and functions. This vocabulary is limited and a single image may be used to represent several things at once. This is what Freud called condensation. For example, a dream of urinating may express a real need to awaken and use a urinal. The same image, however, may also represent that you are "pissed off" at someone. Dreams of urination or other toilet scenes could also be an attempt to assimilate feelings associated with toilet training.

Much depends on the feeling tone of a dream. A dream of defecating accompanied by a feeling of relaxation may indicate that you are holding on to something that you need to let go. If the same dream is accompanied by feelings of disgust or being "dirty" a different set of meanings is suggested.

It is important for you to learn to understand your dreams as *messages* that you send to yourself. Think of them as communications from someone who knows you very well and is trying to tell you something you need to know. It would be a shame to ignore such messages.

Understanding your dreams does not necessarily mean interpreting them. Interpretation *translates* dream imagery into verbal language, a process that reduces your non-verbal imaginal creation to a set of verbal conventions. While there may be value in interpretation (it can help you articulate your personal story and realize a need for action) it is often more important that you assimilate your dreams *emotionally*. This means *facing* your feelings rather than dodging them through some intellectual exercise. What use is it to possess the words that *explain* your neurotic fears while you remain enslaved by them?

There has been some interest lately in learning to become self-aware while dreaming. This is called "lucid" dreaming and has been studied as a way of manipulating dreams from "within". Some have even called this "dream yoga". Yoga's use of dreams is a complex topic to be discussed later (see Chapters VII and VIII). You need to know, however, that by trying to alter the course of a dream you may distort or obscure its message.

The value of dreams is that their imaginal process circumvents social restrictions to express your deepest emotions. Altering a dream's content converts a dream into an egocentric fancy. This may make you feel like a shaman, but it may be counter-productive to the aims of yoga. It is better to leave your dreams alone until they have been fully expressed, and only then work with them using conscious imaginal techniques.

According to modern yoga psychology dreams are classified as fancy and not as sleep. The term "sleep" is reserved for that state of consciousness in which dreams do not occur. Modern sleep researchers identify this as "deep" sleep, a state characterized by EEG slow waves suggesting a suspension of cerebrocortical processing. Dreaming sleep on the other hand is identified by the appearance of fast-wave activity (indicating active information processing) and rapid eye movements (REM).

The ancient yogis did not have access to EEG technology. They noted that a person awakening from sleep sometimes reported dreaming and at other times reported "nothing". In the latter case when the sleeper "looked back" into the sleep period they drew a "blank". They could, however, report feeling either rested or tired.

Presumably, these feelings were construed as evidence that they (1) had slept well or poorly, and (2) were conscious of the quality of sleep during sleep. They also seem to have reasoned that since consciousness must have persisted during sleep the report of a "blank" after awakening evidenced the entertainment while asleep of an image of "nothingness" or "non-existence".

Such an image was assumed to represent a preponderance of the quality of inertia during deep sleep. The presentation of an image of "nothingness" was consistent with the idea that the primary task of mental process was to construct and present objects to consciousness. Consciousness, identified with Pure Being, must always be present and non-being cannot possibly be.

To me, this way of thinking lacks parsimony. It seems much simpler to assume that you have no experience at all during deep sleep, but having slept well or poorly, make a post-sleep attribution based on how you feel after awakening. In other words, if you feel good upon awakening you say to yourself that you *must* have slept well, etc.

This then is not a matter of direct perception during sleep, but one of inference after the fact. As for the assumed non-interruption of consciousness during sleep it makes more sense to follow William James and view your waking consciousness as "knitting over" the blank in order to preserve your sense of personal continuity.

Actually it doesn't matter much how you conceive of what happens while you sleep. The truly important question is "who" is it that needs to maintain a sense of personal continuity during deep sleep. To whom is this continuity important? Who has all these supposed experiences of non-being, feeling rested, or not rested? These questions will not be answered through verbal arguments or EEG tracings. Only practice will lead to an "answer".

We have examined five classes of experience or knowledge: right knowledge, wrong knowledge, fancy, sleep, and memory. No matter how many ways your knowledge and experience may be classified, *all* forms are ultimately *constructions* of your own mental process.

This is not a claim that there is no world "out there" to impinge upon your senses. Pragmatic testing suggests that there is. Whatever that "real world" world may be, however, you experience it only through the medium of your senses and mental process. In other words, what yoga psychology calls the world of "nature and experience" refers to your cognitive constructions.

Some might despair that such a position is too solipsistic in that it leaves each of us constructing our private little "realities". I don't think it does. Life teaches us very quickly that there is much in experience over which we have no control, and that wishing doesn't make things happen unless we take appropriate action.

The important point is that since the world of Nature and experience is a cognitive construction you can always find some avenue through which to take responsibility for the quality of your experience. You may not always be able to control events, but you can exercise considerable choice in how you view them and respond to them. You do not have to make a career of misery.

Also, keep in mind that *all knowledge and experience are entirely ephemeral.* Nothing in nature and experience can be regarded as stable or secure. It follows that if you would know true security you must look not to sensory-perceptual experience, but to the *source* of experience.

No mental process can provide you with absolute freedom from Misery. Every type of experience/knowledge can be a bearer of pleasure *or* pain. Right knowledge can include bad news. The most delicious fancies eventually wear thin and in their addictiveness cut you off from actual living. You may entertain fond memories, but in the end they bind you to the dead. Dreams, on occasion, may be delicious, but most are troubling and some are nightmares.

Since any given mental process can become a vehicle of misery you need to know how this happens if you hope to learn freedom from misery. Therefore, let us now look at the nature of misery and its manufacture.

5

The Making of Misery

All the classes of experience and knowledge discussed in the last chapter operate with the "I"-thought as root. In other words, you experience your thinking and imagining as "belonging to", or being the "product" of, the "I". You may find it helpful to understand how this egocentric foundation comes about and contributes to the making of Misery.

The appearance of the "I"-thought marks the emergence of self-consciousness. The "I"-thought, also called the ego function, divides your perception into perceiving subject and perceived object. This separation of subject and object initiates all dualistic thinking and is a critical part of the construction of your experience. It leads you to perceive yourself as an individual observer separate from the world of observed objects.

This sense of separation is a delusion! The perceived dualism of subject and object is a construction of your own mental process and belongs entirely to the world of virtual reality. Nonetheless, this delusion of separation dominates your thinking and will continue to do so until you take steps to free yourself.

According to modern yoga psychology, the delusion of separation has its roots in the separation that occurs at your physical birth. Whether or not the delusion is a necessary consequence of your physical birth is not an issue here. The critical point is that the origins of the delusion are sufficiently early in your development that they constitute a pre-verbal foundation from which all subsequent mental process proceeds. This means that the delusion of separation is a tacit assumption/feeling held at your deepest unconscious level.

The perception of separation functions as a prime motivator of your behavior. This experience may range from fear of loneliness and rejection to the terror of disintegration that underlies schizophrenia.

The experience of these symptoms can be encompassed by one word, "insecurity". A feeling of insecurity is the primary expression of the perception of separation and is the great hobgoblin of human existence. Insecurity is the emotional shadow of perceived separation.

As a highly dependent and impressionable infant you could not possibly escape the shadow of separation. It was destined to seep into every crevice of your life. It was then to be projected into shadows on the nursery wall, the dark at the top of the stairs, and the absence of caretakers. When insecurity entered your dreams it turned them into nightmares.

Prior to the arising of the "I"-thought you did not feel such insecurity. Separation had not yet come into your experience to cast its shadow upon your inner world. Not only did you not originally perceive yourself as separate, you did not perceive yourself at all. You were not self-conscious. You simply were, seamlessly, at one with all Being.

Before your birth, in the "maximum security" of your mother's womb, your every need was met so automatically and swiftly that you had no awareness of need or want, and hence no awareness of one who needed. Your conscious existence was devoid of desire for you experienced no lack or danger. You did not know insecurity, affliction, or disconnection. Having no such problems you had no need for any self-conscious mental process with which to solve them. You had no need for "mind".

It is not clear whether this secure state began to shatter at birth or shortly before. It is possible that prenatal events altered your mother's and therefore your body chemistry in ways that produced feelings of separation. The important thing is that your womb-like security did come to an end.

The physical separation from your mother at birth had to be a shock. If you were fortunate, the shock was quickly soothed-over and the rupture more or less "re-sealed" through the responsive attentions of loving caretakers. This re-sealing restored your sense of oneness and security, for a time.

Eventually, the comings and goings of your caretakers made it impossible for your life to remain "seamless". The feeling of safe oneness became harder and harder to maintain. The nipple did not always magically appear whenever you felt hunger. Physical holding was not always forthcoming on demand. You came to experience periods of want and desire.

The repeated sequence of a felt need, lack of satisfaction, desire, and then finally the appearance of your caretaker from "somewhere" helped build an image of that caretaker as an "other" who was not always "here". You gradually came to perceive the "somewhere" as "somewhere else" or "not here". This took time to develop, but it reinforced your feeling of separation.

Knowing precisely how the feeling of separation arose is not as important for you as discovering how it operates in your own psyche. You must put aside theory and look within yourself. This may be difficult because it requires that you face your fears and anxieties rather than deny them. If this sounds like a repeating theme to you, get used to it. It will come up again and again.

In my experience, the best way to overcome feelings of insecurity, or any other negative feelings, is to face them squarely. Avoidance will only produce a psychic "cramp". If you can accept the presence of the feelings it becomes possible to begin to "see through" them to their felt root. This root is not historical, but ever present. I refer to the "I"-thought. The delusion of separation and the feelings it generates are rooted in the emergence of the "I"-thought. This is true for all.

With the rising of the "I"-thought the shadow of separation fell across your mental process. Insecurity and a deep feeling of disconnection became the "bogeyman" of your existence. As a consequence anxiety drove you to organize your mental world around the search for security.

Your search for security can be viewed as an obsession with re-connecting to something you feel is missing in your life. This is felt, however vaguely, as a problem to be solved. Problems are the domain of mental process. Your mind thus becomes devoted to seeking sources of security.

The arising of the "I"-thought occurs concurrently with the arising of the world of nature and experience. The world "out there" becomes identified as the source of "others", especially those who appear and disappear in the course of meeting (or trying to meet) your infant needs. The world of nature and experience is thus perceived as your primary source of security, the place to which you turn for relief from anxiety and the fulfillment of desires. As a result you seek to overcome the shadow of separation through connection with the world "out there" and fall prey to the "lure of the senses".

It is through your senses that you learn to look outward for connection. Your senses, the "doorways" to the "world out there", become established (in your view of things) as the means of seeking security. You learn to look outside of your self for all the objects of your desire.

Besides, whenever you look within you risk confronting the shadow of separation and the anxiety it generates. The lure of the senses combines with the avoidance of anxiety to make the "outer world" appear a place of great safety and security. As soon as you turn from your inward shadow toward the world of experience you feel relief.

This feeling of relief is a powerful motivator to keep you focused on the external world of nature and experience. This world becomes the territory in which you seek security. Your mental process thus becomes highly focused on predicting and controlling natural events, as well as working overtime to conjure images of familiarity, safety, and comfort.

All study of the world of nature and experience (i.e., philosophy, natural science, and technology) is at base an attempt to construct security through prediction and control. We all have a low tolerance for uncertainty and tend to fear what we cannot control. After all, nature can be dangerous. At base, science and technology are attempts to pull the teeth and claws from "red" nature. You may talk about "curiosity drives" or a "will to explore", but beneath it all is the need to predict, control, erase uncertainty, and be secure.

Insecurity is also the prime motive behind magic and religion. These, in their own way, are also "technologies" of control. The methods differ from those of science, but the goals are the same. Magic and religion seek to influence nature through supra-natural means, i.e., by circumventing, or in some cases simply denying, the laws of nature.

Religion normally includes appealing to some "higher" power to take one's side against life's adversities. Most prayers, therefore, are supplications for a deity's help in securing safety or success. The religionist feels more secure believing that a deity is on his/her side. All a person needs to do is determine what that deity requires in order to become the recipient of its largesse. This invocation of a power or being *higher* than ourselves conceptualizes the ultimate source of security as essentially "other".

Natural science seeks security through the prediction and control of natural events. This leads to dependence for security on the development of technologies. Such an approach seems rooted firmly in the idea of nature as *external*, i.e., belonging to the world of the object.

Both science and religion make it very easy for a person to seek security *outside* of one's self. Whether it is dependence on the intervention of a deity or the application of a technology, both positions lead us away from looking within ourselves. Yoga psychology holds that the efforts of natural science, magic, and religion all share a turning toward something *external* in order to find security, and that the problem with such outward seeking is that it rests on a fundamental delusion. That is the delusion that the ultimate source of security lies outside of us rather than within.

Yoga teaches that the solution to the problem of insecurity rests with looking within for deep self-knowledge. That search alone can bring about the recognition of your own True Self-nature. No amount of magical appeal, scientific study, or worship can substitute.

The primary reason for this, according to classical yoga and modern yoga psychology, is that scientific efforts and most religious efforts are principally mental and conceptual. That is, both operate upon a conceptual foundation of one form of dogma or another. This makes the search for security in science and most religion a product of primarily mental (largely linguistic) effort. Yoga asserts that the truth of the matter is that deep self-knowledge requires mental silence, and mental silence cannot be produced by conceptual and linguistic exercise. What this means is that security is not to be had among the workings of the mind either through the disciplines of science or religion.

Please note that I have said "most" religion depends upon mental and linguistic work. Clearly there are those in the history of religion who have and do practice silent prayer. If such prayer is truly silent it can slip free of the conceptual entanglements of theology and other linguistically dependent operations. Genuinely silent prayer merges, I believe, with yoga meditation.

The act of seeking security in the external world of nature and experience through either conceptual-linguistic mentation or prayerful supplication effectively turns your back on your True Self-nature. When you look either outward or upward you look away from your True Self that is inward.

You would be correct to object that terms such as "inward", "outward", and "upward" are conceptual, i.e., pure verbalisms. I use them only to contrast the attentional foci of those who seek for solutions to the problem of insecurity through attachment to "realms" that cannot provide any lasting solution. By "inward" I refer to that "direction" of inquiry that gets you to the root of your insecurity. That root, of course, does not have a spatial location. The use of a spatial metaphor is convenient to allude to your looking for answers in the wrong place.

Looking for answers in the wrong places and thereby turning your back on the right place, is called, in yoga psychology, "Ignorance". This refers to an *active* ignoring of Reality and not an absence of some special knowledge. The Sanskrit word for Ignorance is *avidya* and means literally "not seeing". Thus Ignorance is turning a "blind eye" to Truth.

Ignorance is the primary source of all human misery. Once Ignorance takes root in your mind the other sources of misery follow like flies to a dung heap. These other sources are the forms that Ignorance takes as it extends its influence over your mental process and inhabits the shapes of your knowledge. These sources are: Egoism, Desire, Aversion, and Clinging to mundane reality (i.e., the Fear of Death).

Egoism, the first source of misery to spring from the root of Ignorance, begins when the "I"-thought (the ego function) becomes identified with your body. This is a delusion of ownership of "your" body, its actions and experiences.

Once the "I"-thought is identified with your body you speak of "my" body, "my" thoughts and actions, "my" feelings, "my" experiences, etc. You feel that bodily pleasures and pains happen to "you" or are "yours". It is Egoism to feel that you are the author or owner of the body's thoughts and actions.

Identification with your body severely limits your frame of reference. Your experience becomes body focused and body referenced. You think that things really are the way the body and its senses present them. This is the egoism of actuality, entanglement with the body, its senses and actions.

Egoism extends into the virtual world as well. In fact, egoism owes much of its formation and functioning to fancy and memory. Without fancy and memory you would not be able to construct much in the way of a personal identity.

The photo album of your personal history is constructed of fancy and held by memory. Each photo represents some conceptualization that you call "your own". Without it you cannot possess your personal narrative and say, "This is who I am". This identity is largely virtual, a bundle of dead photos strung on the string of the "I"-thought. The resulting "necklace" is a burdensome chain.

Please understand that Egoism involves ownership of both actual and virtual reality processes. Some think that by merely switching from the virtual to the actual, i.e., enhancing "direct" sensory awareness, you can free yourself of egoism. This is not so. Actual experience is still experience and a product of mental process. As such it can be infected by Ignorance as much as virtual process. There is no true freedom until mind's inherent silence is realized.

Yoga psychology calls identification of the "I"-thought with the body, its actions and its experiences, the "Great Knot". The "knot" is an image of entanglement and constriction, an interruption of the natural flow of spontaneous living.

Your body is part of nature and in your identification with it you become a prisoner of all the forces and changes that operate within it. Of particular importance is the biological struggle for both individual and species survival. Survival is a major biological project, a dominating theme in nature. When you identify with the body you become survival's slave.

Concern with survival intensifies the anxiety that arises from the delusion of separation. It intensifies your outward orientation and the lure of the senses. You become more "tied off" from your inward sources of natural creativity, the open and clear awareness that is your heritage of Being-Consciousness. Your life becomes constricted as you focus ever more strongly on your felt need for security. Life becomes a struggle.

The untying or cutting of the Great Knot is a primary goal of yoga psychological training. Inward study will reveal how and where you tie your own knot so that you will know where to cut with the sword of discipline.

Blinded to your True Self-nature by the lure of the senses and concern with survival, your life becomes preoccupied with seeking pleasure and avoiding pain. Preoccupation with seeking pleasure is called Desire and is the third major source of Misery after Ignorance and Egoism.

The enjoyment of pleasure, in and of itself, does not pose a problem. Trouble begins when pleasure becomes a point of attachment and ownership. Trouble begins when your ego says, "my pleasure", and becomes absorbed with seeking and grasping for more.

From the yoga psychological point of view, Desire is self-torture. Desire implies lack of fulfillment in that you desire what you do not have. Desire involves focusing on what is missing in your life. You see your glass as half empty rather than half full. Thus you become trapped into seeking an impossible fulfillment. You pour and pour, but your glass always seems half empty.

Seeking eventually leads to another source of Misery called Aversion. Once you become entangled with Desire you inevitably come to worry about the loss of objects of desire. You become obsessed with avoiding loss.

Aversion is not limited to entanglement with loss. Aversion includes entanglement with all forms of pain and unpleasantness. The main thing, however, is that Aversion leads to preoccupation with avoidance. Such preoccupation seriously constricts your ability to enjoy life. Aversion is a source of Misery.

Bear in mind that it is the entanglement with pain and loss that causes Misery. Pain and loss themselves are not Misery. The entanglement grows out of Egoism's identification with experience so that you actually begin to define yourself accordingly. When pain and loss become an integral part of your personal story they are hard to let go. You think that your story is really you and to give it up seems tantamount to non-existence.

The same, of course, is true of Desire. Egoism breeds attachment to both pleasant and unpleasant experiences because of your identification with the body. You think you are your body, therefore you think you are what your body experiences, pleasant or unpleasant.

Desire and Aversion do not apply only to gain and loss of material goods and bodily pleasures. You can also become attached to spiritual experiences and feel loss and frustration when they are not forthcoming or don't last long enough.

What is the "dark night of the soul" if not the withdrawal agonies of those who have had some kind of peak or spiritual experience, but can't get it back. The problem, of course, is that even spiritual experience is still experience and just as ephemeral as any other kind of experience. You will not find lasting salvation in any sensory-perceptual experience.

To identify yourself with experiences binds you to Egoism, Desires, and Aversion. Rooted in the "I"-thought and the insecurities of perceived separation, you sentence yourself to a narrative dominated by clinging, seeking, and avoiding. You embrace the egocentric games of competition and comparison, praise and blame, victory and defeat, gain and loss, etc. You learn to fear failure and rejection, and your storyline becomes a constant struggle to achieve and acquire.

Of course, if you fail to achieve according to your material expectations you might choose an underdog role and construe yourself as a victim, one of the oppressed and downtrodden. This may allow you to avoid guilt for not "getting ahead" in the world. You could even reframe yourself as a seeker or mystic whose "spiritual achievements" are invisible and not available for public accounting.

What you need to keep in mind is that the affliction of Desire includes craving for both material and spiritual attainments. Seeking and searching for either sets you up for miseries. Material and spiritual greed are two sides of the same miserable coin.

Entanglement with games of Desire and Aversion eventually reaches a point where the thought of letting any of them go seems like personal annihilation, the end of your story. You feel that you must keep struggling else you will fall into the abyss. Here you encounter the fifth source of Misery, the Fear of Death.

The Fear of Death is the "flip side" of your clinging to mundane reality. This includes your attachments to both actual and virtual realities. The Fear of Death is your fear of letting go of nature and experience. You cannot conceive of a state of no experience, it appears so vacuous and frightening. This is why so many turn away from classical yoga's invitation to silence in favor of forms that appear less threatening, e.g., sensory "scanning", guided imagery, relaxation, and the like.

Egos do not easily contemplate their own non-existence and will grasp at anything that seems to offer some way to cheat death. Denial of death takes many forms ranging from theologically sophisticated to the adolescent assumption, "I'm young and it can't happen to me". Whether you escape into belief in an afterlife or via the distractions of thrill seeking, sex, or drugs, the aim is to avoid facing your own personal death.

If you turn to religion or philosophy for consolation you are still seeking to avoid death. Most religions promise some kind of after-death survival either in a rewarding paradise or another try at life via reincarnation. Many who cannot accept either of these alternatives still seek salvation through mystical experience. This, however, only encourages your dependency on experience.

Yoga psychology asks you to face the prospect of your own death and discover what it actually amounts to. You must learn to look within and face the shapes that fear takes in your psychophysical life. Study these and learn their ways. This, and not avoidance, is the path to spiritual freedom.

Classical yoga describes nine psychophysical obstacles that arise from the sources of Misery. These are what you actually experience when you are in Misery. They are your body of Misery. I refer to disease, languor, laziness, indecision, carelessness, sensuality, misconception, missing the point, and instability.

Disease, or "dis-ease", refers to a loss of equilibrium that may be expressed by overt bodily symptoms and signs or more subtle emotional processes. In either case your psychophysical system is stressed and you suffer accordingly.

Languor and laziness might seem to be the same, but they are not. Languor is the feeling of a lack of energy or enthusiasm. You lack any feeling of motivation and find it difficult to take pleasure in things.

Laziness, on the other hand, refers to the felt presence of inward "heaviness" or resistance to movement. There are things you want to accomplish, but you feel weighed down and held back.

Indecision refers to the inability to make up your mind. Frequent changes of mind and inaction may reveal themselves in hesitation and awkwardness. It does not take much imagination to see how concern for the consequences of action can play a role here. Fear of failure, humiliation, and loss of status can all breed indecision.

Carelessness impairs both thought and action. It can manifest as illogical and/ or uncritical thinking, and is the hallmark of the intellectually lazy. Carelessness in thought can make you appear stupid. Carelessness in action leads to awkwardness, accidents, and generally poor performance.

Sensuality is attachment to objects of sensory pleasure, and includes both lust and gluttony. Sensuality is a spawn of Desire, but ought not be confused with it. Desire is entanglement with pleasure of all kinds both material and spiritual. Sensuality focuses on physical pleasures.

Keep in mind that yoga psychology makes no absolute distinction between physical and spiritual realms, but views them as part of a single continuum of experience. Many people eschew physical attachments, but then take pride in their pursuit of intellectual or mystical "achievements". They fail to understand that Desire is Desire whatever the object. A craving for spiritual experience is still craving.

Misconception is the entertainment of a false view of something, i.e., the misinterpretation of sensory information. It also includes mistaking virtual reality for actual reality, and mistaking either for Absolute Reality.

Missing the point means failing to attain concentration, i.e., not being one-pointed or present-centered. It includes looking in the wrong place for something or taking a wrong direction. When you miss the point you do not focus on the task at hand. In discussion and debate, for example, you cannot follow an argument to its conclusion, and fail to "get the point".

Instability refers to an inability to remain concentrated. You can attain concentration, but are unable to keep it up. As a consequence you become mentally unsteady.

Concentration is essential in yoga psychology. In fact, yoga may be defined as concentration. Concentration is essential to doing anything well whether spiritual or mundane. You cannot acquire skill without concentrating on instructions, demonstrations, and actual practice. Whatever you try to accomplish you must focus your attention on what is relevant and let go of what is not. This goes for physical, intellectual, and spiritual pursuits. If you want to hit a home run in any field you must keep your eye on the ball.

All the obstacles may be experienced singly or in combination. If you study yourself you may notice that one obstacle often turns into another. Frequently they coexist. What is important is that all obstacles are manifestations of the infection of your mental process by Ignorance, Egoism, Desire, Aversion, and Fear of Death.

When obstacles beset your life it is easy to feel that you are a victim. Try not to fall into that trap, however. A victim attitude will get in the way of your facing obstacles and learning how to see through them to their roots in the sources of Misery.

When you discover an obstacle in your life don't despair and lapse into blaming and whining. Instead, try to see each obstacle as an opportunity to learn something about your self, a revelation of what you need to work on.

Facing obstacles requires the mastery of certain skills (see next chapter) and lots of patience. Misery is rooted in long standing habits and those habits will take time to dismantle.

The current operation of each obstacle in your life has roots in karmic seeds that were sown in the past. It is the fruit from these seeds that you must face in your present life. As you do so you will gain more understanding of karmic cause and effect. That knowledge will enable you to deal more effectively with current fruit, in addition to preventing the fruition of seeds yet to sprout and not sowing further seeds.

Let us review. The obstacles that you experience as misery arise from the sources of Misery. These sources are Ignorance (not seeing/recognizing your True Self-nature), Egoism (identification of the "I"-thought with the body and the felt ownership of its processes), Desire (hankering after both material and spiritual pleasures), Aversion (preoccupation with pain and loss), and the Fear of Death (clinging to ordinary reality, i.e., nature and experience). Of all these sources Ignorance is primary. All Misery flows from Ignorance.

Whatever forms your search for security may take, know that they are rooted in Ignorance and that Ignorance operates only by means of your own mental process. Think of Ignorance as a virus that structures your mental process to its own ends.

You must understand two fundamental truths. One is that the sources of Misery can only operate and propagate through mental process. Therefore, if you can learn to quiet your own mental process Misery will have no field of operation and will dissipate.

The other truth is that there is no mental process that, in and of itself, provides absolute security or freedom from Misery. Mental process manufactures the world of nature and experience and cannot be divorced from it. The entire operation of mind and nature constitute a web of interlocking processes all of which are transitory and cannot offer any kind of abiding security. There is no safe haven in mental process and therefore none in experience. Even right knowledge can be subverted by Ignorance.

This does not mean that you should reject all experience or not enjoy experience. The entire purpose of experience is enjoyment. Enjoyment is the natural heritage of your True Self-nature. Know, however, that there is no security in enjoyment because all objects of enjoyment are part of the process of nature and experience and thus ephemeral. By all means, enjoy, but do not cling!

If you truly understand the manufacture of Misery as described in this chapter, you will realize that it points directly to the path you must follow in order to get free of it. This is the real promise of yoga psychology, and it is time for you to investigate this path.

6

Concentration

This chapter moves you from theory to discussion of actual practice. If you have not done so already there is no better time than right now to check out the meditation exercise in Appendix A. If you do not engage in actual practice what follows will remain just more verbiage.

Yoga psychology defines practice as any *effort* to steady your mind. I draw your attention to the word "effort". Let no one tell you that effort is not needed, at least in the beginning. Effort is necessary to counter your long-standing habits of thought. These habits mean that any instruction to simply "go with the flow" will leave you circling at the starting gate. Practice requires effort.

The primary technique of practice is concentration. Concentration means bringing your mind to *rest* on a single point, e.g., a visualization, mantram, or the natural rhythm of your breathing (see Appendix). I emphasize "rest" because too often one-pointed concentration is presented as something forced and unnatural.

One-pointed concentration is perfectly natural and can, if practiced properly, lead you to making a *pleasing* connection of your mind with its object. If you think of the flow of your mental process as a series of *moments*, at every moment your mind is perfectly concentrated on some object. The problem is that old habits, driven by karmic seeds, control your concentration in the interests of Ignorance and turn your mind toward one of three unproductive states: the *fickle-minded, distracted,* or *sluggish.*

In the *fickle-minded* state your mind is unable to stay with one object for more than a few moments. Although it may be perfectly concentrated on object "A" one moment, it shifts to object "B" the next moment, and then very soon to "C", "D", etc. The fickle mind cannot stay put and such a state is not helpful to the practice of yoga psychology.

In the *distracted* state your mind does not jump from one object to the next, but becomes absorbed with an object other than the one intended. For example, you want to rest your mind on the rhythm of your breathing, but a sexual fantasy comes up and gets you off track.

Such a fantasy clearly arises as a distraction from within. Other distractions, however, may appear to arise from without. Sounds from the street or the apartment upstairs can become such "external" distractions if you allow them to "get to you".

These sounds are not inherently distracting. They pose a problem only if you attach meaning to them. If, for example, you hold to a preference for some "perfect" meditative atmosphere, e.g., the near silence of a Zen garden, your preferred atmosphere will conflict with what is actual. The gap between what is and what you prefer will cause you irritation. It is, of course, the internally generated irritation and not the street noises that create distraction. In this sense, all distractions are generated internally.

In the sluggish state your mental process becomes dominated by inertia. You may experience confusion, torpor, and a desire to sleep. Sleep is a well-known "enemy" of meditation. When your body needs sleep it will try to take it. This means that if you do not want sleep to disturb your meditation you must get enough at the appropriate times.

The fickle-minded, distracted, and sluggish states are of no use to the practice of yoga psychology. Only two states are useful and those are the *one-pointed* and *empty* states. The empty state will be discussed towards the end of this chapter.

The one-pointed state occurs when your mind is fully focused on its chosen object. Its importance cannot be overemphasized. No task, spiritual or otherwise, can be accomplished with skill unless you concentrate on it. Any athlete, artist, writer, chess master, mathematician or other problem solver will tell you that this is so.

The concentrated mind not only permits the application of skill it frees you from conflict. Any conflict requires your having at least *two things* in mind at the same time.[1] When your mind is one-pointed conflict is impossible.

When you first begin to practice meditation you will no doubt find that your mind tends to be dominated by one of the three non-productive states. This is because when meditation is not a well-established habit, other habits will intervene. You may experience distracting fantasies, fickle-minded darting about, and a tendency to drop off to sleep. Do not despair. Be patient with yourself.

---

1.   Strictly speaking having two things in mind at the same time is not possible. Conflict is probably best viewed as involving a continuing alternation between two or more thoughts.

When you find yourself in one of the non-productive states don't waste time chastising yourself or otherwise cursing your mental condition. That will only make it worse. When you become aware that your concentration has broken simply return your attention to the chosen object. You may need to do this many times, but try not to despair or give in to feelings of failure. The concepts of success and failure are irrelevant. Instead, know that your awareness of having drifted from concentration means that your meditation is slowly ripening.

This brings you to the importance of pairing the practice of concentration with the cultivation of *desirelessness*. Desirelessness and practice are the two arms of action (*kriya*) yoga and a vital part of yoga psychology.

Desirelessness is defined as the *feeling of inward mastery that comes when you have let go of seeking for material and spiritual attainments*. Don't enter into meditation with the idea that you are going to "get" something or "achieve" something. Meditation is not about achieving; it is about letting go! It is better to practice simply in order to practice and let the results take care of themselves.

If you must have a goal in mind think of realizing silence. When you are truly silent your mind will no longer be tortured by clinging to goals and achievements. Try to approach your practice not as seeking or doing, but as being.

Until such time as you can truly let go, you will most likely find that most of your meditation practice involves learning how to deal with perceived distractions. You may construe distractions as arising either from without or within, but all distractions actually arise from within.

For example, you may feel that you are distracted by sounds coming from the street. Indeed, if you live in a noisy neighborhood such sounds can prove difficult at first. You may come to notice, however, that it is not so much the noise itself that distracts, but your *irritation* with the noise that is the problem.

I remember beginning my own practice while living in a small studio apartment in New York City. My ideal images of practice at that time had me sitting in a Zen monastery in medieval Kyoto or some equally exotic place. The sounds I heard in my city apartment were not those of breezes through pine branches or frogs jumping into ponds. I had *preferences* and the sounds of the city *conflicted* with them.

After much practice I came to let go of this romantic image and just sit quietly listening to the constant low drone of the city. This city sound eventually became very comforting to me and substituted well for the sounds of ancient Kyoto. Eventually I accepted that a dropped garbage can was a good substitute for the sound of a frog jumping into the pond. Was this "advancement"?

No, because I had only let go of one preference for the establishment of another. I went from finding the city noises irritating to savoring their calming drone. The drone became associated with occasional inner quiet and in so doing I gave it importance. I began to desire a certain "drone-silence-feeling" and made it the mark of a "good" meditation. Do you see what occurred? I merely moved from one attachment to another. So much for my cultivation of desirelessness!

When you find yourself getting entangled with any object or experience other than the one chosen for meditation (e.g., your breathing) let it go by returning to the chosen object. Do not even bother to label it as a distraction for that introduces value. If you are resting your mind on your breathing try to get the feeling of "breathing away" your entanglement as you exhale. Keep letting go.

To let it go means just that: no embrace, no rejection, and no entanglement. Simply return your attention to the chosen object and let whatever came up go its own way. Should it remain, let it alone. Don't trouble with trouble. You are not seeking perfection. You are not seeking anything. Take your time. Be patient.

Some texts describe "stages" or "levels" of concentration. These usually depend either on the nature of the meditative object or on the kind of "distractions" that arise, e.g., "gross" or "subtle" objects, etc. You might think of these "levels" in relation to the various processes or functions described in the chapter on mental emergence.

A precise description of these levels is not really important. What is important is that by staying with your chosen meditation object and maintaining a *pleasing* connection you automatically subject each type or "level" of mental process you encounter to the clear light of *discriminative wisdom*. This wisdom enables you to recognize each aspect of your mental process as belonging to the realm of nature and experience and being entirely ephemeral. Thus you learn to discriminate that which is unreal (i.e., transient) from that which is Real, i.e., your True Self-nature.

When such discernment takes place you will find it easier to let go and disentangle yourself from your attachments to nature and experience. There is much from which you must disentangle yourself. Think of it as learning to let go of all that is ephemeral and not Real, or as a quest to find your True Self. Ask of everything that arises, of each layer of mental "stuff", "Is this lasting and dependable?" or "Is this what I am truly?" No one can answer these questions for you. You must do the work.

As you practice you will learn to disentangle your self from many "layers" of mental process. You will find initially that much of your mental process is occupied with ordinary discursive thinking. This includes all thought processes mediated by language, e.g., internal conversations with your self and virtual others regarding interpersonal issues, problem solving, rehearsing, reworking arguments that did not go well, and all manner of just plain worry.

Much of this rumination involves your ongoing attempts to construct and maintain your personal narrative. When things don't go according to your preferences or images of yourself you retreat to your virtual world and "rewrite" them. You may, for example, need to construct or reconstruct various explanations (theories, hypotheses) in order to make anomalous experiences fit your beliefs and expectations. All of this is done in the interests of preserving the security of your egocentric self-image.

You may discover that much of what comes up in your mind are fancies that attempt to make your life appear more successful, less boring, etc. Sometimes these fancies can lead to creative solutions to problems, but too often they only serve as substitutes for needed action. The temptation to hide out in your virtual world is always there.

The constructing and maintaining of your self-image involves more than words, however. Your self-image involves your non-verbal experience of your body and the fact that you identify yourself with it. That is, you think that you are your body, and this belief is a major underpinning of your self-conscious life. It is the essence of Egoism.

Much of your body-centered conversation involves things like looking in the mirror and trying to see yourself in the best possible light. You may try to talk yourself into seeing someone in much better shape than you truly are, or it may involve the reverse process in which you judge yourself to be an absolute mess. In most cases fancies of competition and comparison are involved and they do nothing but promote Misery.

As you go about constructing your personal narrative and trying to see yourself according to your expectations it is important to realize that these expectations are usually not explicit. More often than not they lurk in the background as unconscious "templates" shaping your experience. One of the aims of concentrative meditation is to bring these assumptions into the open where they can be exposed to your discriminative wisdom. You begin to see their lack of truth.

Many of these underlying assumptions include a personal list of unconscious *directives* and *injunctions*, i.e., do's and don'ts. A directive might be something like, "you must always be a 'nice' boy/girl", or "you must always strive to 'get ahead'". An injunction, on the other hand may take a form like, "I will never be happy" or "I can't do math."

A good many of these mind structuring "commands" come from things your parents or other authorities said to you when you were too young to question them. You took them as gospel. As a consequence of this social "hypnosis" they became severely limiting parts of your personal story, themes of Misery rather than of Joy.

To realize your inherent freedom from Misery you need to learn to "see through" these "rules" and "lies". This is part of learning to discern the actual from the virtual, and the Real from the ephemeral. It is how you wake up from the hypnotic sleep of Ignorance.

As you become aware of the role played by internal conversations, unconscious assumptions and rules, you are better able to let them go. As you let them go you become aware of even "deeper" assumptions and beliefs. Many of these are not so much personal as they are transpersonal, i.e., they are part of your cultural heritage (a form of karma). Since these are shared and unconsciously supported by others in your culture they may be even harder to discern and question.

These transpersonal assumptions work unconsciously to form the foundation for your more personal mental processes. Among these are those that Jungian psychologists call "archetypes". Archetypes have been described as "templates" that shape personal experience according to largely bio-cultural imperatives. They include powerful mental tendencies to structure experience in terms of basic ideas such as "God", "the mother", "the sanctuary", "the hero", etc. These and other themes appear in myths and also in dreams.

More fundamental than archetypes are the structuring elementals of time, space, and cause. These are perhaps the best examples of so-called "subtle" mental processes in that they operate at the most unconscious levels and may be the most difficult to appreciate. Nonetheless they exert a huge influence on your experience. In fact you most likely cannot conceive of experience without them.

The overwhelming tendency is for you to take time, space, and cause for granted and never question their reality. You think of them as absolutes. That, however, is an error. They are pure fancies, conceptual constructions of your mental process.

We know that time, space, and cause are relative and conceptual (i.e., ephemeral constructions of mental process) because they are so easily altered through pharmacological intervention and by environmental manipulation. For example, basic alterations in the perception of time, space, and cause are common in descriptions of drug induced hallucinogenic experience. In addition, many purely behavioral experiments have shown that our daily perceptions of the world are clearly constructed out of our own assumptive mental processing rather than objectively representing a "world out there".[2]

Concentrative meditation eventually throws these basic mental categories into relief where you can see for yourself that they are not absolute. This kind of "seeing through" is an important aspect of yoga psychological re-education. Remember that the basic task in concentrative meditation is for you to discern the Real from the not real, the relative from the Absolute, i.e., the ephemeral from the lasting. Ultimately this means learning to recognize your own True Self-nature amidst all the social constructions and miseducation that have been heaped upon you.

After seeing through the relative nature of time, space, and cause you may experience a profound Joy. This feeling arises from the realization that you are inherently free of these limiting dimensions as well as all other social and linguistic constructions. As you realize this, however, you need to be aware of several very important things.

One is that the Joy that you feel is an *intrinsic* part of your creaturely nature and is not dependent on objects. In other words, Joy arises from *within* rather than coming from outside of your self. The mental construction that you can actually *take* joy from objects is a conceptual error. In actuality you have intrinsic Joy within and experience it when you *put* that joy into your daily living. This realization frees you from your long-standing dependence on specific objects for joyous experience.

The experience of Joy does not signal the end of your yogic work. Joy, however wonderful, remains part of the world of your experience and is ephemeral. Do not confuse Joy with "enlightenment" or absolute "liberation". It is a step in the right direction, but not the end of the journey.

The experience of "unalloyed" Joy can become a real sticking point. You can become attached to the experience and through that attachment launch yourself into yet another cycle of misery. You may have heard of the "dark night of the soul" suffered by mystics. The "dark night" occurs when someone who feels s/he has "seen" God or been otherwise blessed no longer feels that blessing. They pray and pray, or meditate and meditate, but get nothing back from it. Prayers are no longer answered and blissful experience cannot be repeated. They feel bereft and abandoned.

---

2.   I am thinking of the experiments reported by W. H. Ittelson and F. P. Kirkpatrick in *Scientific American*, 185 (August 1951) 50-55.

This, of course, is the classic consequence of attachment to any kind of experience. It is well known to drug addicts and alcoholics the world over. Their language may not contain the "exalted" verbiage of the mystical aspirant, but the psychology is the same.

All experience, however sublime, comes and then goes. Nothing in the realm of nature and experience lasts forever. This is why attachments and dependencies can only lead to misery. It does not matter if you play the game at a high spiritual "altitude". Misery is still misery.

You must let go of Joy. Do not seek it. Forget about it. Let the guru proselytizers and academics talk about Joy and bliss all they want. In order to finish the work of yoga psychology you cannot afford to linger over and count your achievements.

This brings you another key question: just *whose* achievements are these grand and glorious experiences? Who are you who seek bliss, transcendence and transformation? Who quests for Truth? This brings you to the "I"-thought that is the root of all thought and thus the foundation of all the mental processes you have thus far "seen through" and let go.

All of your seeing through and letting go is equivalent to rejecting each "level" or aspect of your mind and experience as constituting the "real you". By continuing to apply yourself to the concentrative meditative process as you "see through" each "layer" of mind you, in effect, have actually been engaging in the equivalent of questing for the source of your "I"-thought through all the regions of your mind.

It does not matter that you may not have conceived of meditation that way. To some extent it does not matter how you conceive of meditation as long as you engage in practice accompanied by desirelessness. The latter is important because some conceptualizations are sufficiently romanticized and mystical to puff your ego into viewing them as "attainments". The cultivation of desirelessness reminds you that there are no attainments, only letting go.

You could think of your course of meditative seeing through and letting go in terms of practicing the dead pose (see Appendix A). Once you have allowed your attention to rest on the natural rhythm of your breathing, get the feeling that you are breathing into each and every part of your body starting at the very tip top of your head and working slowly and carefully down to the ends of your toes. As you "breathe into" each part of your body you in effect bring your attention to bear on that part and become fully aware of it. As you exhale you try to get the feeling of breathing the part away, just letting it go. You might even visualize the part floating off into space and disappearing. To breathe into a part and become aware is to "see into and through" it. As you realize that it is not the absolutely real you, you let it go as you exhale. It is best that a teacher talk you through this exercise the first few times before doing it on your own.

Once you survey your entire body and let it go as being "not-Self" you can turn your attention to your mental life. As mental process rises up you can attend to it by "breathing into" it and then "breathing it away". None of it is really your Self. This includes all "layers" of your mental process including the feeling of Joy that arises from genuinely letting go of limitations and restrictions. Especially joyous is the gradual realization that you are not your own body!

Look at that last statement, "*your own* body". This feeling of owning "your" body is egoism pure and simple. You must ask, therefore, "who is this 'I' that feels and thinks that it owns this body?" To do this you need to hold the "I"-thought as your object of concentration. Then, as you hold to the "I"-thought, seek its source.

Only by holding to the "I"-thought can you ultimately "see through it" and let go of it. Letting go of the "I"-thought is letting go of all mental process and with it, your identification with the body. When you focus on the "I"-thought you see through the "great knot" that ties you to the ephemeral world of nature and experience. Focus upon the "I"-thought frees you from birth and death.

According to the late sage Ramana Maharshi, the source of your breathing and the source of the "I"-thought are the same.[3] That is, when you simply allow your mind to rest on the natural rhythm of breathing in and out you are, psychologically, pursuing the source of the "I"-thought. By practicing what Buddhists call "mindfulness of breathing" you seek the source of the "I" however you may conceive of it. Your practice will be on target even if you have no conceptualization of it!

Yoga psychology calls all concentration upon a given object "meditation with seed". This has several meanings. It can refer to the fact that your concentration has a specific object or focus, e.g., the vocalization of "Om", the visualization of a light inside your head, or the natural rhythm of your breathing.

Meditation "without seed" on the other hand is a practice in which there is no specific object. This occurs when the object of concentration drops away and leaves nothing but clear, empty space.

"Without seed" also refers to a condition in which all karmic seeds (or residue) have been "burned up" and can no longer sprout. Prior to this, any empty space

---

3.   See *Sayings of Sri Ramana Maharshi*. A. R. Natarajan (Ed.) Ramana Maharshi Centre for Learning, Bangalore. 1966.

cleared by the dropping away of a concentrative object was quickly filled by content generated by remaining karmic seeds.

When your practice finally frees you of all karmic residue the clear open space of your "original" mind is manifest. This is the absolute silence that permits the recognition of your True Self-nature. Conceptually it is the "end" of your mind.

You could call this end of your mind "crystal clarity", "open space", "emptiness" or whatever you please. You must discover for yourself this Truth beyond words and concepts. To this end I prefer the term "emptiness" because it offers less temptation for you to conceive of yourself as seeking, attaining, and trying to identify some special state. Remember that your True Self-nature is not an experience or a state. It has no identifiable characteristics.

"Attainment" is best conceived as not knowing that you have attained. Or, as the *Daodejing* might put it, "Those who are aware of having attained have attained nothing, while those who are aware of attaining nothing have truly attained." It follows that practice, apart from the effort to steady your mind through concentration, is silence and not seeking. You might think of it as simply Being your Self.

There is still a further meaning of "without seed". When your actions are egoless they spring from an empty, or non-clinging, mind. Such actions do not *sow* further karmic seeds. When you act out of clear "emptiness" your actions are automatically desireless and do not create karmic consequences. Such actions are spontaneously dexterous and appropriate to their circumstances.

When your actions flow from desirelessness they are free of egoistic motives and thus truly benevolent. There is no concern for "virtue" and "goodness". Self-righteousness has finally been slain. Your deeds are benevolent without your knowing it, unselfconscious expressions of your True Self-nature. This is Supreme Naturalness.

A metaphor comes to mind. Consider the gradual clearing of the sky following a storm. Initially all is dark as rain clouds obscure the blue sky. Eventually the clouds become lighter and small patches of blue can be seen. As the clouds slowly drift away the sky becomes even clearer and more brilliantly blue. Finally, there is nothing but a bright blue clarity that you recognize as having been there all along. Then, because you have cultivated desirelessness, you let go of the blue and realize an empty clarity free of objects.

The path of practice (effort to achieve mental steadiness or clarity) requires patient persistence. It may help you to remember that your True Self-nature is already here and that practice involves removing mental obstructions to that recognition. In this context "distractions" are always opportunities to let go and rid your self of another "gray cloud".

Never forget that Practice must be coupled with Desirelessness. The idea of "progress" and attainment is foreign to meditation. It is egoistic and does not apply. Your work is not to "get somewhere" in order to "be this", "become that", or experience something special. Your task is to let go and be. Remember, you can always let go a little bit more.

7

Supports For Concentration

The discipline of concentrative meditation is not practiced in a vacuum. There are many "accessory" disciplines that must be practiced in order to minimize distraction and find your strength for concentration.

Yogic tradition divides these supports into "outer" and "inner" disciplines. Outer disciplines include ethical and "moral" training as well as the management of interpersonal relations. The point of such training is to avoid conflict. If either your inter- or intra-personal life is in conflict it will impair your attempts to practice.

There is no concept of "sin" in yoga psychology. There is only the awareness that there are processes that cause misery and interfere with practice. Thus, although texts may refer to "ethical" or "moral" principles, these should be viewed simply as *training rules* for spiritual practice.

In addition to training rules students practice physical postures and breath control. Together with the training rules these constitute the "outer" discipline. As such their practice is considered supportive of the "inner" discipline, i.e., concentrative meditative practice. Concentration was described in the preceding chapter. This chapter will focus on elements of the "outer" discipline starting with the training rules.

These rules include both restraints and observances. You are advised to restrain from (1) doing harm, (2) lying, (3) stealing, (4) lusting, and (5) greed. Each of these five restraints is intended to avoid attitudes and behaviors that conflict with the aims of yoga psychology.

Restraint from harm is fundamental and as close to a "moral law" as yoga psychology gets. Harm refers to any kind of physical, psychological, or spiritual injury done to yourself or another. Simply put, causing harm never does any good. It sets in motion chains of events that only cause pain, conflict, and more harm. Ask yourself, "What good comes from causing injury to another or myself?" In all its forms, e.g., vengeance, punishment, rage, abuse, etc., harm only causes misery.

Students of yoga psychology are advised to practice *benevolence* toward others in order to avoid doing harm. Benevolence is incompatible with harm in that it involves acts that support and nourish others. It also counters the egoistic tendency to push one's own agendas to the detriment of others. Benevolence includes providing psychological and emotional support whenever the opportunity presents itself.

Adherence to truth entails being honest in all your dealings with others and with yourself. If you are true to yourself you will be better able to be truthful with others. This means that overcoming self-deception is a major requirement for the student of yoga psychology.

It also means that you must face "what is". Maintaining clear presence of mind in all situations is the foundation of truthfulness. Meditation helps you develop presence of mind. To be fully present is to stay on track in the here and now. To stay on track is concentration. Facing "what is" is part of "seeing through" falsehood and delusion. Facing "what is" is letting go of your lies.

Practicing Truth combats Egoism. Egoism, working through Desire, Aversion, and the Fear of Death, attempts to maintain its own image of self and in so doing builds a framework of deception and lies. The ego cannot tolerate living in a world where it is subject to birth and death. Egoism cannot accept the actuality of the death of the body because Ego is *of* the body. Ego thus becomes a master of denial and other defensive ploys.

Students of yoga psychology do not steal, i.e., they do not take what isn't theirs. Stealing is motivated by Egoism and Desire. When you steal you put your wants ahead of others and risk harm to others. Since stealing reinforces Egoism you harm yourself by reinforcing the machineries of Misery.

Restraint from lust does not mean abstention from sex. Lust is egoistic greed focused on sexual gratification. It is a form of grasping that makes sex an instrument of Ignorance. Since sex is basic to the biological life of the body it easily becomes a vehicle of Egoism, Desire, Aversion, and Clinging. When that happens the sexual urge is easily subverted to interests beyond its natural purview. This causes no end of trouble. You must ask yourself if you seek sex to feel safe. Do you confuse sex with acceptance, power, control, or ownership? If so, you are clearly treading the path of Ignorance and Misery.

Because sex involves powerful physical feelings it lends itself to being an absorbing distraction from pain and displeasure. Sex can be used as a kind of analgesic, a way to avoid facing "what is". Unfortunately this makes sex a vehicle of Aversion. (For more on sex see chapter IX on *tantra*.)

Restraint from greed also aims at limiting egocentric thought and action. Greed represents entanglements with objects such as money, food, power, prestige, etc. In all cases of greed impulses that might otherwise rise and fall of their own accord become neurotic compulsions that defy satisfaction. Material, social, and spiritual possessions are pursued in the delusion that they can provide absolute security. They cannot. The only consequence of greed is Misery.

It is important to remember that it is *attachment and entanglement* with objects that constitutes greed. There is nothing intrinsically wrong with having money, property, and social influence if you put them to benevolent uses and do not depend on them for things they cannot deliver. Since money, property, and power are ephemeral it is critical that you learn to use them without getting entangled. Then, when inevitable loss occurs, you will avoid Misery.

Similarly, there is no inherent virtue in poverty. True poverty, in the spiritual sense, refers to non-attachment and the ability to let go. True poverty refers, in part, to an attitude of non-grasping.

Too often, those who harbor a sense of failure over a perceived lack of material goodies in their lives hide behind a show of spiritual poverty. That is, having little or no aptitude for coping in the material world they are eager to advertise their "spiritual" possessions. Outwardly they claim that due to their spiritual status they have no desire for material things. Inwardly they are as grasping as the next person.

The restraints are the "don'ts" of yoga psychology (even though some are better explained as "do's"). The *observances* are the "do's". Again, it is important not to view these in terms of "virtue" and "vice" (remember, there is no concept of sin in yoga psychology). Like the restraints, the observances are training rules that, if followed, take your life out of the path of Misery. The observances are cleanliness, contentment, austerity, study, and spiritual devotion.

Cleanliness, sometimes called "purity", refers to both external and internal practices. External cleanliness includes bathing, following a healthful diet, and other common sense observances of bodily hygiene. The point of these is to promote good health and avoid the distractions of illness.

External cleanliness also includes maintaining "clean" relations with others and with your environment. You should avoid contaminating your relationships with competition and comparison, shaming and/or blaming, labelling, manipulation, and other behaviors that cause injury, defensiveness, and generally destroy relationships.

External cleanliness, however, depends upon internal cleanliness. It is difficult to have good relations with others if you are riddled with doubt and negative self-imagery. Defensive projection can lead you to see these negatives as belonging to others. Internal cleanliness includes recognizing and seeing through such processes and then letting go of them.

Support and encouragement (the instilling of courage) of others need to begin with your self. As always it is the sources of affliction (Ignorance, Egoism, Desire, Aversion, and Clinging) that comprise the spiritual "dirt" you must keep from dominating your inner life. Then you will be in a better position to avoid passing the "dis-ease" on to others.

Internal cleanliness includes the cultivation of a clear mind that can look into itself fearlessly. A clear mind is free of egoistic striving and defensiveness, and does not let itself be controlled by a fear of consequences. In the end, the pinnacle of internal and external cleanliness is the mind of crystal clarity well established in an uncomplicated calm.

The practice of *contentment* is learning to be satisfied with *what is*. This includes being satisfied with what you have and not seeking more than you need. It also extends to letting go of unproductive reactions to situations. For example, no amount of yelling and cursing to yourself or out loud will clear the road of stalled traffic and "bad" drivers, or reform a detested "city hall." To take effective action without adding to your karma of Misery, your mind must be clear.

This does not mean that you should cultivate a Pollyanna attitude toward adversity. What is important is to realize that when you act out of frustration and anger you will usually make things worse rather than better. Contentment is a state of mental poise that is not disturbed by circumstances of any kind.

Practicing *austerity* is closely related to practicing contentment and involves letting go of your attachments. This pertains to both external and internal possessions as well as personal relationships. The practice of austerity requires that you discern the difference between your needs and wants. Many so-called needs turn out to be mere wants, i.e., manifestations of Desire or Egoism.

Do not forget that the practice of austerity includes cognitive as well as material and spiritual possessions. If you want to cultivate a clear mind let go of attachment to views and opinions. Ask yourself if everything rattling around in your head is really that useful. Do your beliefs lead you into paths of Joy or Misery? Do you cling so tenaciously to your views that you cannot listen attentively to other opinions? Have you allowed yourself to become the prisoner of your intellectual preferences?

Austerity entails letting go of the *inauthentic* as well as the superfluous. Perhaps your burdens are "gifts" from others. When I was much younger I used to argue a politically conservative line that was an unthinking echo of my father's opinions. I was "inhabited" or "possessed" by his opinions. When I started thinking for myself I came to realize that many of his ideas were inconsistent with my own experience and feelings. I realized these views were a burden I needed to let go.

The *Bhagavad Gita,* an important text of yoga psychology, declares that it is more blessed to *fail* at your own duty than to succeed at someone else's. To be yourself you must listen to your own "drummer". Amidst the noise of societal pressures this is not easy. Still, if you would truly enjoy your brief life, you must discover and pursue your own duty.

It is not a question of success or failure. True enjoyment comes from the *pursuit* of what is truly meaningful to you. This is because it activates your personal potential or "duty-nature". This nature is not absolute; it is ephemeral and temporary. Nonetheless it represents an expression of absolute Truth.

Here is another word on austerity. Yoga psychology teaches that you travel best when your hands are free (i.e., not grasping or holding on). So, as you work on yourself, bear in mind these words of my own teacher: "Once there was a man, though many thought him mad, the more he gave away the more he had."

The requirement of *devotion* has been interpreted in many ways. Usually it is rendered as "devotion to the lord". "Lord", according to modern yoga psychology, is your True Self-nature or the image of one who has succeeded in recognizing his/her True Self-nature.

Such a person is free of birth and death, no longer experiences separation, and stands as a beacon of Truth. This is what it means to be "lord" of the universe. It is an inspirational image or sign pointing your way to Practice and the cultivation of Desirelessness. It advertises the Reality of deliverance from Misery.

Devotion to such an image speeds the way to your freedom. Devotion need not imply a conventional religious view. For yoga psychology devotion means adherence to *practice* and *desirelessness* rather than to some power or force conceived as "higher" or "other".

I need to make yoga psychology's position clear on this point. Yoga psychology is devoted to the recognition of your own True Self-nature. It asserts that you have a True Self-nature, but refuses to say what it might be because you are to discover or recognize that Truth for yourself. If you must conceptualize your True Self-nature view it as "pure being", i.e., it simply *is*.

You might go on to speak of it as absolute, independent, unconditional, and without form. The problem with this is that it is not an "it". Better to admit that your True Self-nature is inconceivable, i.e., cannot be conceptualized in any way.

This "inconceivable" nature also rules out conceptualizing the "lord" as any kind of a deity. The "lord", as previously mentioned, is simply an individual who has recognized his/her True Self-nature and thereby realized freedom from Misery.

Most people who practice religion worship a personified deity. They require a personal form for it is difficult to worship or pray to a formless abstraction, e.g., "the absolute". In those cases where a relatively abstract "force" or "great spirit" is addressed there will be found "lesser" deities of a more anthropomorphic form. Even when animal spirits or powers are addressed we endow them with human qualities. It is very hard for us to give up projection.

Usually a personal deity is conceived as a super parent of some kind. This projection of a parent image brings with it the feeling that the deity is "higher" and "other" than the worshipper. The worshipper is conceived as "helpless" and the deity as possessing powers of nurturance, reward, and/or punishment.

Such conceptualizations of a deity as a "higher" power may serve, psychologically, to promote surrender and dismantle egoistic striving and grasping. This is the primary role of the "higher power" in twelve-step programs such as Alcoholics Anonymous.

Yoga psychology is more than willing to use worship of a deity in this way. However, if such conceptualized deities and powers are regarded as absolute truth or unquestionable doctrine they represent idolatry. Idols (as opposed to memory aids or meditation props) become foci of grasping and dependency, and as such are antithetical to the process of yoga.

How the use of such conceptualizations and imagery is managed in one's practice is for a student to work out with a teacher. The avoidance of idolatry is, eventually if not immediately, necessary.

No one has stated the difference between yoga and religion better than Geraldine Coster in her book *Yoga and Western Psychology* (see Appendix B. Suggested Readings). Coster argues that there is a profound *practical* difference between yoga and religion. With yoga the image of a deity may be used as a focus for concentration. The point of using the image is to enlist relevant emotions in order to *intensify concentration*. In yoga the goal of concentrative absorption is primary while devotion to the deity is a means to that end. In religion, on the other hand, devotion is primary, and concentration is practiced for the purpose of intensifying it.

This means that from the yoga psychological perspective there will come a point when the image of the deity must be let go. Yoga aims at mental silence, i.e., formless or objectless meditation. When the deity is paramount, the sensory image of that deity may become an obstacle. In terms of the observances, when devotion becomes idolatry it violates the practice of austerity.

In addition to devotion to practice and the realization of your True Self-nature you are advised to *study*. This includes any activity that sharpens your Self-understanding and supports Practice. It can range from reading books and attending talks by people who actually have something meaningful to say, to fearless self-examination. The latter is particularly critical.

Self-examination calls for you to identify and let go (not reject) all in yourself that is not real. This task runs from questioning your cognitive assumptions to the practice of Self-inquiry. Self-inquiry may begin with using the question "Who am I?" as a concentrative focus and the move to seeking the actual source of the "I"-thought. The latter may be seen as the "highest" form of devotion.

Study in yoga psychology includes being mindful of the quality and dynamics of your interpersonal relationships. It is within relationships that your constructed social self finds definition and your defensiveness seeks targets for projection. Other people play an important role in how you come to view yourself. How you judge yourself is often revealed in your judgments of others. When you find yourself being critical of others stop and ask if you are not actually finding fault with some aspect of yourself. After all, your ego will find it easier to judge others than itself.

As you do this bear in mind that ego is a mental process and not an entity. To learn to let go of egoism you need to understand how it operates and infiltrates your daily relationships. You may long to view your spiritual life in terms of wrestling with some cosmic angel, but it is more likely (and more useful) that you need to wrestle with your mundane judgments and attitudes.

Your interpersonal relationships, viewed either from the outside or the inside, are part of the human jungle. There will be potential entanglements wherever you turn. You may try to flee the conflicts of your family or the commercial world for the serenity of the monastery, but you will then have to contend with the conflicts of that environment.

People are people wherever you may find them. Gather more than two people together and you will find all the natural tendencies towards cooperation, competition, disagreement, alliance formation, favoritism, and a host of political games. None of this is "good" and none of it "bad". The intensity of human conflict varies with the maturity of those involved, but you will still have to cope. Self-study helps you see through it, keep your ego out of it, let go of it, and thus better negotiate the tangles.

To help you minimize inter- and intra-personal strife yoga psychology offers, in addition to the restraints and observances, the *practice of contraries*. This cultivates attitudes and behaviors that are contrary to those that promote conflict and cause Misery. Included are the cultivation of *friendliness* towards those who are happy, *compassion* to those who are in pain, *complacency* toward virtue, and *indifference* to vice.

Practicing *friendliness* to those who are happy counters envy and jealousy, and helps overcome the conditioning of a culture dedicated to competition and comparison. If your neighbors win the lottery congratulate them and support their joy. It is better than stewing in envy.

Believe me, you *can* learn to do this without being a hypocrite. If you feel envy of someone's good fortune recognize your true feelings, admit them to yourself. If you then say to the person, "I am so happy for you" know that it is a lie. If, on the other hand, you were to say, "that is great for you" it would not be a lie. It really is great for them no matter how you feel about it, and you will have taken a small step toward weaving a fabric of friendship.

The practice of *compassion* towards those who are suffering counters feelings of helplessness, hopelessness, and fear you may feel towards those who are sick or injured in body or mind. The feeling of aversion in reaction to the suffering of others often comes from the fact that their suffering penetrates your denial of the actuality of pain and mortality. You are reminded that your defenses are not fool proof, and that all human individuality ends in old age, sickness, and death.

You may find that you cannot turn compassion on and off like an electric light. Instead compassion arises spontaneously when avoidance and other egocentric attitudes have been let go. Prior to that you may try to fake compassion, but it is not clear that this is really helpful. Some argue that you may have to "fake it" before you can "make it", but I find that sentiment troublesome. It invites dishonesty.

Perhaps it is better to admit a lack of compassion and the presence of "inappropriate" feelings to yourself and accept that you are not a great saint after all. (The sooner you do this the better.) Then do what you know to be right even if your feelings would move you in the opposite direction. This is not "faking" compassion, but practicing the contrary to "wrong" action.

The practice of *complacency toward virtue* may seem unusual if you have been taught that virtue deserves praise. As the cliché goes, however, virtue is its own reward. This means that truly good deeds (i.e., benevolence) flow naturally from a clear mind and do not require rewards to make sure they keep occurring.

If you seek rewards for your acts you are practicing Egoism. Ask yourself, when you do "good deeds" and are not recognized for it, do you feel slighted? You may think that you are giving of yourself, but by thinking that you deserve recognition you reveal the lie. Genuine giving seeks nothing in return. In real giving you let go of the gift. This is the difference between giving and deal making. With a deal there is always a *quid pro quo*. In giving there is letting go.

Rewarding virtue belongs to the game of praise and blame and is rooted in dualistic thinking. Dualistic thinking arises from the delusion of separation. It is born of Ignorance. Yoga psychology teaches that you need to free yourself of dualistic thinking.

The practice of *indifference to vice* may be hard to grasp at first. You have probably been taught to look down upon and even fear people whose behavior is judged vicious. The problem is that the standards by which societies judge behavior as vicious are variable. What is a vice in one culture (or sub-culture) may not be a vice in another. More often than not such judgments boil down to personal and cultural *preferences*. That is, you call what you like a virtue and what you don't like a vice.

From the standpoint of yoga psychology the concepts of virtue and vice entangle you in dualistic thinking and nasty (vicious?) games of blame and shame. Blaming often reflects an egocentric desire to feel superior to others. Given the human propensity for projection blaming usually involves assigning your own worst faults to others. Beware that the stones you cast don't turn into boomerangs.

Most often it comes down to learning to let go of the vexations that arise when you or others act in ways contrary to your preferences. Some people, for example, are virtually unable to ride in a car without finding fault with the way other people drive. They are fond of pointing out how everyone else runs stop signs, fails to signal turns, etc. Such judging wastes a lot of energy and if you do it while driving you are not really paying sufficient attention to your own driving job. Instead of finding fault with others it is better to keep your eyes on the road.

If you would be the keeper of a clear mind, let go of concern over virtue and vice. Do not enshrine egocentric preferences with labels of "right" and "wrong" or "good" and "evil". It only perpetuates dualism and foments Misery.

When most people hear the word "yoga" they think of postures and stretching exercises. This is because the majority of those who claim to teach yoga appear to limit their practices to physical health and fitness and pay only lip service to genuine spiritual concerns. Very few, I suspect, are trained to be spiritual teachers.

This is not to say that you shouldn't take a class that teaches only postures. Such classes can be of physical and even psychological benefit. If your teacher is sufficiently skilled s/he can teach you to sit properly. That after all is the primary aim of posture work. You may, however, need to look elsewhere for true spiritual instruction. For example, there is a well-known instructor of postures who takes meditation and spiritual instruction from a Tibetan Buddhist lama. This instructor's own teacher had offered nothing in that domain.

The real problem with many yoga classes is that, lacking any attention to your *inward* life, postural training often leads to stronger rather than lesser identification to your body. In other words, postural study without spiritual discipline may perpetuate Egoism.

In yoga psychology posture training is conceived as *supporting* inward meditative discipline and letting go of attachments. The primary long-term goal of postural training is, therefore, the cultivation of mental silence, clarity, and attitudes conducive to both practice and desirelessness.

The more immediate practical aim of posture work is the attainment of a comfortable position for meditation. Normally this is a cross-legged sitting posture, but meditation may be practiced while standing, lying on your back, sitting on your heels or in a straight-backed chair, or while moving in a prescribed manner (e.g., taijiquan). The essential point is that your body should be comfortable and not become a source of distraction.

When the sage Ramana Maharshi was asked what he considered to be the most useful yoga posture he answered, "concentration!" In other words the inner work of concentration is paramount, and any posture than helps you concentrate is good. It also suggests that sitting in a "perfect" lotus posture without concentration is not really sitting at all. It is *performing*. It may look great for the centerfold of some yoga magazine, but it misses the point.

All proper work with postures involves concentration. The correct practice of any posture calls for you to be fully present to (focused upon) your body-in-the-posture or on the particular bodily area where letting go is required. If you are doing a posture and thinking about what's for lunch or how slim and esoteric you look you are not really practicing yoga psychology. The point is to cultivate concentration and mental clarity, not to perform in a circus or be the star of a video.

Ideally, the meditation posture should be effortless. If your knees, ankles, back, or other parts of your body ache and keep announcing themselves you will have difficulty attaining mental steadiness. A calm, steady, and effortless posture leads to a calm, steady, and quiet mind.

Unless you are uniquely gifted, however, effort will be necessary in the beginning. Physical habits associated with non-yogic states of mind need to be let go and this can take time. Persevere, however, and you will be able to perform the necessary postures with an attitude of inward steadiness and calm clarity. Be patient with yourself and keep at it.

In a very real sense posture is about *attitude*. In yoga psychology postural attitudes are practiced to induce and strengthen psychological attitudes. For example, postures help you develop "wind", "backbone", and "guts". Each of these can be associated with an attitude. Wind refers to control of your breath and will be discussed below. For the moment you should know that proper breath control requires an upright posture. Learning to sit with your back straight, but not rigid, is essential to yogic breathing exercises.

You may guess that "backbone" and "guts" refer to the qualities signified in colloquial language. Backbone refers to being able to "stand tall" in the face of adversity. It implies courage or heart. If your back is strong you will not bend easily to manipulation. You will not be one of those who are always "bending over backwards" for everybody.

At the same time you want to develop flexibility. It is one thing to stand tall and "stay the course", but you must also be able to bend or twist when necessary. Knowing the difference between firmness and rigidity, as well as when to be immovable and when to dodge artfully, requires training.

It also calls for the development of discernment. As the song goes, "You gotta know when to hold 'em and know when to fold 'em." Clarity, discernment, strength, firmness, and flexibility come together with proper training and self-discipline.

If you have "guts", or "intestinal fortitude", you will not allow fear to distract you from your duty. It doesn't mean that you never feel fear, but that you do not let it become an obstacle. You are able to maintain concentration and act decisively even when fear rises. Whatever the task, the better trained you are, the more you will be able to let go of fear and act with a clear mind. When your mind is clear your skill and courage manifest in action that is spontaneously appropriate to present circumstances.

Many postures require that you relax certain muscles in order to perform the posture properly. This relaxation is part of learning to let go. The "trick" is to relax the muscles without causing undue strain and risking injury. Yogic posture training is not a "bop 'til you drop" proposition. Concentration, care, and caution are recommended.

Whenever you encounter resistance or strain don't force the issue. Instead bring your attention to bear on the specific feeling of resistance in your body and get the feeling of breathing into that place. As you breathe in and out feel that you can actually move breath into the relevant areas. Then, as you exhale, try to get the feeling of letting it go. With practice and patience your muscles will relax and the posture becomes easier.

When you are practicing postures keep in mind that your primary purpose is to support meditation and letting go. Use posture training to help you let go of attachment to your body rather than strengthen that attachment. This calls for putting meditation's inward work ahead of concerns about your physical appearance, competition, or comparison.

Posture training helps prepare you for working with your breathing, and breathing directly affects your mental process. Being able to sit comfortably with a straight, but not rigid, back facilitates your breathing. If you sit slouched over your lungs will not have enough room to expand fully and you cannot take a complete breath.

You need to be able to sit erect with your back straight, but relaxed. You can use your breathing to help with this. As you breathe in try to get the feeling of lifting out of the small of your back. As you do, feel your chest rise and your shoulders roll back. Let your shoulders relax rather than assume a military "brace". As you breathe out feel yourself letting go, but don't let yourself fall into a slouch.

Breath is closely associated with the play of energy in your body and mind, and is part of what some call the "subtle body". However you conceive of it there is no doubt that slow, deep, and regular breathing has a calming effect on your emotions and mental process. It is very hard to quiet your mind when your breathing is irregular and/or shallow.

It is important to learn to take a complete breath. If you are like most people your present habit is to use only a small fraction of your true vital capacity. A simple technique is to focus on your exhalation and observe its outward flow. Towards the end of the outflow tighten or draw in your abdomen and "squeeze" out as much breath as you can. Do this gently, but firmly. Never force anything. When your lungs feel empty, relax your abdominal muscles and let your inhalation proceed naturally. As you inhale you may notice that your abdomen extends. Let the inhalation continue until you feel the breath rising into your chest area. Do not force yourself to breathe in more than feels natural to you. Let the inhalation take care of itself. At the top of the in breath hold your breath for about two seconds and then permit yourself to exhale. Again, follow your exhale and end by "squeezing" it all out, etc.

If you have any medical conditions such as asthma, emphysema, high blood pressure, or heart disease you should consult your physician before taking up any kind of yogic breathing. There are many techniques of breathing in yoga, and you should be able to find a procedure that will work for you. Some methods are more complicated and forceful than others and could exacerbate certain conditions. You should be especially cautious about techniques involving holding your breath. If you experience any pain or discomfort while doing a breathing exercise stop and consult with your teacher or physician before continuing. In any case it is always best to practice breathing exercises under the supervision of a qualified teacher.

A good way to start on your own, however, is simply to observe your breathing without trying to control it in any way at all. Such mindfulness of your natural breathing rhythm is really more of a meditation than a breathing exercise, but it will gradually deepen and regularize your breathing over time and is a good place from which to branch into other breathing approaches should that be suitable. Mindfulness of breathing can be very calming, however, and you may not need any other technique.

Traditional yoga discusses breath control in terms of inspiration, expiration, restraint, and "motionless suspension". At a superficial level "inspiration" simply refers to the in-breath and "expiration" to the out-breath. At a more subtle level these terms refer to the *inward feeling* of a "need" or "urge" to inhale after expiration and exhale after inspiration. It is useful for you to become familiar with these feelings by observing the natural movement of your breathing. It will help you approach control without falling into harmful forcing.

The terms "inspiration" and "expiration" are also associated with the movement of "spirit" or bodily energy. "Inspiration" refers to being inspired, i.e., filled with "spirit", animation, or "aliveness". A person who is inspired pursues tasks with concentration and vigor.

"Expiration" or "expiring" can refer either to relaxation, letting go, or death. We say a person "expires" when s/he dies. The final out-breath is truly a letting go, the end of the struggle. The ancients (and more than a few moderns) believed that the final expiration at death signaled the actual departure of one's spirit.

In breathing meditation you are advised to get a feeling of letting go whenever you breathe out. While this obviously helps you relax physically, it is also the practice of letting go of your body and all related attachments. Such practice helps you become familiar with the silence of death.

Do not think of this as a gloomy or morbid practice. You do not know what death is. You only know what you imagine it to be, and those imaginings are constructions rooted in fancy. If you cling to life you will fear death and naturally think of it in sad and gloomy terms. Because of your identification with the body death seems like the end of everything for you.

However, who is this "you"? Before you fret about your death you really need to know *who* it is that lives and dies. Yoga psychology teaches that asking such a question is far more fruitful than clinging to life through fanciful consolations of an afterlife or reincarnation. Think about it. Why fret over what happens at death when you do not really know who you are this very moment?

With extended practice at observing your breathing you will find that your breath slows naturally without your having to resort to "advanced" techniques. Your breathing may even slow to a point where it seems that you are not really breathing at all. This can lead to awareness of a deep stillness or "space" between breaths and between thoughts. This space is not *caused* by your practice, but is *revealed* by it. It has always been there, awaiting your recognition.

As your mental process slows and edges towards silence you can begin practicing *withdrawal of the senses*. This is turning your attention away from the "outer" world towards the "inner". You use the regular rhythm of your breathing (or whatever focus you have chosen) to "slide down" into your "interior". This is the beginning of self-investigation via concentration. With the training and support of the preceding disciplines (restraints, observances, posture and breath control) you begin the real inward work.

You may wonder if this distinction between "inner" and "outer" is merely conceptual, a fancy lacking actual substance. Of course it is a fancy, but it is a temporarily useful one. While there is no absolute "inside" any more than there is an absolute "outside", the delusions spawned by Ignorance lead us all to think the distinction is actual. The distinction is useful in a relative way until you see through it and let it go.

Understand that direct "seeing through" is not simply an intellectual conclusion reached by a verbally mediated logical process. Logic has nothing to do with it. "Seeing through" refers to a realization that does not depend on words. It is more of an "aha!" experience that occurs when something previously obscure becomes self-evident.

"Seeing through" enables you to let go of your entanglements with the sensory-perceptual world of nature and experience. These entanglements came about when you forgot your True Self-nature and sought to avoid the resulting anxieties of felt separation by seeking security in the world of the senses. This seeking, by the way, helped crystallize your dualistic mental construction of "inside" and "outside".

At a feeling level it began with something like "If I look here I feel great anxiety so it feels better to turn and look the other way". This evolved into the cognitive construction of "a dark and frightening inner world" contrasted with the "hope of safety in nature and experience".

It is much the same as drowning your sorrows in alcohol, drugs, or sex. All are distractions from anxiety and temporarily provide an illusion of comfort and security. It is all part of the play of Ignorance.

Thus you begin your yogic practice entangled with and dependent upon the world of the senses. No doubt it frightens you to conceive of life without your senses. This is your fear of separation. This fear is precisely what practicing withdrawal of the senses is intended to reveal and eventually heal.

Since you must begin where you are, i.e., in the midst of your constructed entanglements, your practice will be construed initially as one in which your attention must turn away from the world of the senses toward the dark and mysterious inner world. This inner world is full of imagined dangers, repressions, fancies, dreams, "monsters" of the Id, and eventually (if you keep at it) silence.

As you practice "withdrawal" of your senses, more and more of this "inner" world becomes "outer". That is, your meditative discipline enables you to face these "demons" and "tame" them. You learn to "see through" this inner "stuff" and realize that it is part of nature and experience, part of your mental construction. You also see that what is constructed is ephemeral and can be "de-constructed".

You gradually come to accept that your attachments to nature and experience cannot "save" you. You realize that you will never find answers to your spiritual questions in the world of experience, be that experience of an "inner" or "outer" nature. You may delude your self otherwise for a while, but your comeuppance will be inevitable. If some natural or human disaster doesn't awaken you there are always old age, sickness, and death to remind you of your bodily limitations. You cannot delude yourself forever.

To turn "within" includes acceptance that the solution to your miseries resides with yourself and not someone else. You recognize that whatever your circumstances your experience of them is determined by your own mental processes. This brings an end to blaming others for your misfortunes and initiates genuine personal responsibility. Your acceptance of this is part of practicing Truth.

Turning within also means that you give up following, imitating, and competing with others. You come to be guided by your own feelings and experience of what works and what doesn't for you. You realize the value of standing firm against pressures to conform and find the courage to follow your heart.

Once you have turned within, your practice becomes largely an inward one. You do not give up the preliminary practices (it is always good to keep up your "ABC's"), but your emphasis is now on the *inner discipline* of concentration proper.

As you know, concentration involves bringing your mind to *rest* on a single point (thought or image). Then your mental process necessarily lets go of all other objects and becomes quiet. When it is quiet, your mind provides no place for Ignorance and its manifestations (Egoism, Desire, Aversion, Clinging to Life) to sink their hooks. Ignorance cannot operate when its field of action has been shut down.

Concentration provides a way of "studying", or becoming mindful, of the nature of your own mental process. This is not an academic or scientific study, but a process of direct seeing-through into the fundamentally ephemeral nature of your mind. It does not matter whether a given process is classified as gross or subtle, exoteric or esoteric. What matters is the realization that *all* mental processes are insubstantial and transient.

The practices of withdrawing your senses and of concentration work together. As you go within yourself aspects of experience that you thought of as "subjective" become "objects" of investigation. These objects are thus exposed to the scrutiny of your developing discriminative wisdom and you "see through" and let go of them. Continued practice, always coupled with desirelessness, allows you to "descend" through the various "strata" of your mental process and realize that none of them constitute your True Self-nature.

Your daily thought processes are not your True Self. Neither are the dark creatures of your unconscious or your deeper cognitive assumptions about space, time, and cause. As you let go of these processes you may feel great Joy welling up from within, but this is not your True Self either.

Through it all you may feel a strong conviction that there is actually a "someone" or "something" lurking behind all your thinking and feeling. This is the "I"-thought, the root of all other thought.

Now, do not take my word for any of this. Look deeply within your own experience. Examine the processes of your "mind" and see for yourself what lies beneath your thinking. If you agree that it is the "I"-thought then take the next obvious step, and seek the source of the "I". This is the quest taught by the sage

Ramana Maharshi and represents the quintessence of the Upanishadic lore. It is what Patanjali called "returning the mind to its source". It is the root koan and represents the culmination of all concentrative spiritual discipline.

The sage Patanjali divided this inner discipline into three main phases. Your passage through these phases represents the process of returning your mind to its source. All of the training and discipline has this as its aim.

The phases are not discrete, but continuous. The first is "fixed attention" which involves focusing your attention on a single object. Initially such practice involves a sense of effort for you are working against the habits of an undisciplined mind.

With continued practice the sense of effort dissolves and fixed attention becomes true meditation. There remains, however, a sense of "I am doing this, I am meditating". You need to let this go for ultimately you are discovering Being as opposed to doing or having.

When the egoistic view is let go meditation gives way to absorption. Absorption implies that there are no longer any intrusions about who is doing the work or what will be the result. There is no longer any concern for the passage of time. Time and space fall away and there is nothing but the chosen point of concentration held firmly in your mind. With continued practice the single point dissolves of its own accord and your practice becomes one of absorption without an object.

Does this mean that only the subject remains? Can the object fall away and there remain a subject, or are subject and object mutually dependent? That is, can there be consciousness without "consciousness of" something? Classical yogic tradition assumes an absolute subject, a *Purusha* or an *Atman*. Buddhist yogis might argue to the contrary, that there is no ultimate subject. This is a largely conceptual issue, however. Ideally, practice should lead to letting go of dualisms and take you to where there is neither subject nor object. Go work on yourself and find out!

After all, is the source of the "I"-thought something your mind can possibly grasp? Grasping, of course, is the primary business of mind. Can a mind grasp its own source? To paraphrase a Zen koan, "Can one hand clap?"

You must do the work and find out for yourself. When you seek the source of the "I"-thought what do you find? Look! Look!

Is this then the end? The old Zen master Dogen (a great yogi in my estimation) said, in effect, that after dropping the last object you must then drop dropping.

8

The Fruits of Practice

The principle benefit of Practice is a clear and silent mind. When your "mind" is clear and silent your True Self-nature reveals itself. It has always been present waiting for you to recognize it.

For mental peace to last, however, you must "burn up" all of your karmic "seeds", i.e., the residue of past actions. Then they will no longer sprout into misery. Your practice of mental stillness creates a calm space in which the seeds may "rise up" and be exposed to the light of discriminating wisdom. Thus exposed you can let them go. To understand this fully you need to know a little more about *karma*.

Karma is the universal law of cause and effect. This law states that for every event there is some causal condition that produces it, and that for every act there are, sooner or later, consequences. Consequences may manifest in either your external or internal environment. Internal consequences may be physical, emotional, cognitive, or all three.

Karma exists in three "states": (1) seeds currently sprouting into consequences, (2) seeds sown, but not yet sprouting, and (3) seeds not yet sown. Current afflictions represent seeds actively sprouting in your present life. It is too late to avoid these consequences, but you can learn to cope with them. Yogic practices help minimize the misery that karma can produce. Well-established habits of concentration and desirelessness can help you let go. Practice (i.e., effort towards mental steadiness) provides "psychological distance" from painful symptoms. It also aids in discerning that these symptoms are not your True Self-nature, but the ephemera of experience. They will pass. With practice and the cultivation of desirelessness they will not return.

Karmic seeds that have been sown, but not yet sprouted, await the conditions that can trigger them. Self-study reveals what those conditions are so you can avoid them. This may involve your taking appropriate action to alter your social and non-social environment. This involves cultivating self-knowledge and learning to assert yourself in responsible ways. You need to learn how to keep your conditioned "habit family" from being reborn in current and future relationships.

Seeds that have not yet been sown need not be sown in the first place. As you learn more about how Misery is caused, you can gain the ability to avoid engaging in actions that sow karmic seeds.

Working to free your self from *karma* is primarily an inward task. It is from within that you can exert the most influence over the quality of your experience. There is often very little you can do to alter the behavior of someone else, but there is always something you can do to change the way *you* react. Consider, for example, when things don't work out according to your preferences do you see it as a personal failure, a catastrophe, a lesson, or a challenge? How you view your circumstances and incorporate them into your personal story sets the stage for both inward and outward action.

Your biological karma places some limitations on what you can do. You cannot flap your arms and fly (of course that didn't stop the Wright brothers). You do not have the sharp claws of a tiger (but you can learn to wield a knife or sword).

The challenge is to study yourself and understand your own duty-nature. Know what is natural for you and what brings you joy in the doing. When you strive according to your own bodily nature it is ultimately enjoyable even though it may take effort and practice to achieve realization. It is even more enjoyable if you can let go of thoughts of competition and comparison. Don't worry about being number one. Instead, learn to "en-joy" your being.

Practice and the cultivation of desirelessness clarify your mind to see through the limitations constructed through social hypnosis. Your imagination is then liberated to reveal new possibilities.

The liberation of your imagination brings you to the threshold of "paranormal" powers, or the *siddhis*. These come to those who are able to practice yogic concentration in a spirit of *non-attachment*, i.e., desirelessness. Without desirelessness the powers easily become a temptation to slip back into egocentric ways, i.e., to manipulate others or just plain show off. It is therefore always good to remind yourself that these powers fall entirely within the domain of experience and are as ephemeral as any other aspect of experience. The special powers are not all that special.

Natural science psychologists tend to dismiss claims of paranormal powers as unproven and wishful hogwash. Parapsychologists counter that there *is* compelling evidence of the existence of paranormal abilities, and they seek to provide experimental demonstrations supporting this view. The natural scientists discount the parapsychological research as flawed, and they all go around "talking through" each other. In my view both sides miss the point.

The parapsychological position seems based on an essentially *religious* faith in paranormal abilities as evidence that the limitations of material and natural existence, i.e., birth and death, can be overcome. I see this as a denial of death just as are beliefs in some kind of afterlife. Popular opinion aside, such beliefs have nothing to do with yoga and yoga psychology.

On the other hand, the natural scientific position, in its dogmatic insistence on "objectivity", goes too far in downplaying the value of human subjectivity and personal meaning. Subjective experience is usually considered too biased and "soft" to form the basis of good research.

In my opinion the dogmatism of natural science throws the baby out with the bath water. While there is no doubt a vast sea of bath water in parapsychology and the occult, I assert that there is also a baby. Let us see if we can find it.

The classical yoga tradition holds that paranormal powers do exist, but are a distraction from real practice and should not be sought. We must ask then, why does the single most important technical treatise on yoga, Patanjali's *Yogasutra*, devote the better part of its third section to such "distractions"?

I suggest that the descriptions of "powers" need not be taken literally as *paranormal* abilities, but may be viewed as metaphoric references to the *imaginal potentials* of a mind freed of Ignorance. Such a view seems to be more in keeping with the internal and psychological emphasis of classical yoga.

The classical tradition lists eight "great powers" or *siddhis* as follows: miniaturization, magnification, levitation, extension, irresistible will, mastery, lordship over the universe, and fulfillment of all desires. Let us examine them as internal *imaginal* aptitudes rather than demonstrable public phenomena.

Consider the powers of "miniaturization", "magnification", "extension", and "levitation". If you practice meditation long enough (e.g., 25 to 40 minutes) and often enough (e.g., once or twice a day), you may eventually notice feeling *as if* your body were expanding, shrinking, or floating off the floor. When focusing attention on a particular body part, e.g., an arm, you may get the sensation that the arm is growing longer. If you *think* of lifting your arm it may actually do so seemingly without volition. Depending on how you deploy your attention, you may feel as if your entire body is expanding out into space and sailing away.

These experiences may be understood as alterations of your *subjective* body image, i.e., the way you experience your body in the privacy of your "inner mind". The profound relaxation and letting go that can occur during meditation include the *loosening of perceptual habits*. This can result in an increased flexibility in perceptual organizing including alterations in how you experience your body's boundaries. For example, the sound of bird chirping "outside" your window may seem to arise from "inside" your own head. There is nothing mysterious or magical in this. It is perfectly natural that the perception of your body, its boundaries and orientation in space, would change as you relax habitual ways of perceiving.

Meditation-induced bodily experiences need not be all that dramatic. Much depends on your expectations and tendencies to dramatize. If you diligently cultivate desirelessness and let go of craving for extraordinary experiences, alterations in body image will more likely seem matter of fact. If, on the other hand, you are a true believer in the paranormal and avidly seek "unusual" experiences you will make more of them. It is in the latter instance that the dangers of distraction are greater.

The real gain of changes in body-image perception has nothing to do with collecting experiences and everything to do with letting go of identification with your body. Your long-standing habit is to identify with your body and construct a virtual world of personal fancy around it in order to feel secure. Meditative awareness of bodily sensations loosens this identification and puts your constructions under the lens of discriminative wisdom. Moreover, it does this under circumstances that minimize anxiety and make letting go easier.

Levitation presents a great symbol. It is an image of "rising above" mundane concerns. Especially important is that as you weaken dependence on your habitual body image you "rise above" entanglement with it. This, of course, means that the great knot is beginning to unravel and lose its ability to bind you to birth and death.

"Rising above" also suggests gaining a new perspective. From "above" you see things differently. This new perspective is not Truth, however, but simply another view. Its value is that it reveals the relative nature of all views. It is good to be free of the "tyranny of views".

Having an "irresistible will" simply means that you can stay the course and not get discouraged. It has nothing to do with "power" over others or your environment. While it may be true that added self-confidence does help you be more convincing to others, the truly important power is inward. An "irresistible will" can withstand distractions and stay on track.

Remember that all "powers" are the result of practice, i.e., the application of steady attention to mental objects, and must be accompanied by the cultivation of desirelessness. Desirelessness is defined as the *feeling of mastery* that comes from letting go of the thirst for material and spiritual enjoyments. This is the real meaning of "power".

"Lordship over the universe" refers to several things. Concentration on any subject leads to knowledge and understanding of that subject as well as to the imaginative application of the knowledge gained. For example, there is no doubt that ancestral human absorption with the behavior of spiders constructing webs contributed to the development of weaving. Native Americans don't revere "spider grandmother" for nothing. She presented their imagination with a great gift. Nature concentrated upon has much to teach us.

The more you can focus your mind, the more you can know. Knowledge is the gateway to effective action. As you concentrate you expand your knowledge of "what is" and dexterity in action follows spontaneously.

"Lordship" also implies mastery. If you are lord you are a master. Keep in mind that this is *inward* mastery, i.e., mastery over your self. There is little to be gained from lording it over others unless you want to sow dissention and destroy relationships. Strive instead to master your inward life through Practice and Desirelessness. Since yoga psychology teaches that your world, your universe, is a construction and projection of your own mental process, inward mastery is mastery over that construction.

Remember also that Desire (a source of Misery) is defined as *hankering* after pleasure. Desire is *entanglement* with pleasure. As a bodily creature of Nature you are going to experience desires. Mastery, according to yoga psychology, is not about achieving an absence of urges or hungers, but learning to avoid entanglement with them. Specific desires are creatures of Nature like the weather. You must learn to cope rather than wish them away or become their puppet. The best course is to let your desires go and don't trouble with trouble.

Please don't misunderstand this. If you let go of a given desire you may well continue to feel it, at least for a while. You do not, however, have to let it *dominate* your thinking. If you try to dismiss the desire or push it away you will be wrestling with it and keeping it in the forefront of your mind where it remains dominant. To let go is to let go, i.e., do not care if the desire stays or goes.

The best way to let go of any one thing is to focus on something else. As with any other kind of distraction a desire may intrude on your mind. You let it go by returning to your intended focus whether it is meditation on your breathing, doing homework, washing the dishes, raking the yard, etc. Let the desire go its own way. Do not try to control it. Let it go! That is the key to mastery and "lordship".

It is the same with "fulfillment of desire". My teacher was fond of repeating, "Once there was man, though many thought him mad, the more he gave away, the more he had." If you can really let go you will feel great fulfillment, not because all your desires have been satisfied, but because *indifference* to them frees you from entanglement and conflict. If you have no preferences you are free of conflict.

When you get entangled with desires it is because you seek to *take* joy from the objects of desire. Practice, however, reveals to you that Joy is not a property of objects, but an intrinsic part of your inner nature. When you can find Joy within you cease depending on externals. This is the meaning of the "fulfillment" of desires.

In addition to the powers already discussed there is another in Patanjali's *Yogasutra*: the "ability to enter other bodies". You might be tempted to see this as the paranormal ability to possess and control the bodies of others, or perhaps the power to shape-shift. You might even begin to harbor an egocentric desire to see yourself as some kind of magician or shaman. To read the aphorism that way, however, would be a misunderstanding.

In yoga psychology the body is conceived as a *vehicle* for action. That is, a body is a temporary configuration of skills, habits, attitudes, cognitions, etc., organized around some intent. Your body, for example, can become a vehicle for the practice of yoga psychology if you organize it by devoting yourself to practice and desirelessness.

Whenever you take on a particular challenge you organize your body accordingly. Your meditation practice or your dreams may reveal that you need to work out some bit of personal *karma* by becoming more assertive rather than allowing yourself to be manipulated by others. Such a revelation is a sign that you need to make yourself into a vehicle for assertion, and put off the "body" of victimization.

Remember that what you call your personality is a mental construction and entirely ephemeral. It is not your True Self-nature and you can learn to change it. No one says such changes are easy, but they really can be accomplished. It is a matter of replacing old habits with new ones. Of course, such "shape-shifting" is difficult if you are attached to a particular way of constructing yourself.

This should give you some sense of the range of yogic "powers" and how they may be viewed as "feats" of a free imagination. I believe this imaginal perspective is much more useful than assuming the powers are objectively demonstrable paranormal abilities.

If you feel disappointed by this interpretation you may need to look at your wish for magical abilities. Ask yourself if you have a craving for such powers and what they might mean to you. Do you wish to deny the insecurities of the flesh? Perhaps your desire for occult abilities is compensation for a sense of inadequacy in your daily affairs. If so, you must find your remedy in actuality rather than fancy. Learn to free your imagination of its fears and come to understand true inward mastery. The practice of yoga psychology will help you find your true strengths and deal skillfully with actuality.

You need to *face* your demons if you want to free your mind of their destructive power. When you face them put yourself in the position to learn what they are made of and thus rob them of their mystery and ability to affect your life. Not only that, it puts you in a position to take their energy and put it to work for you. It is your energy anyway.

For example, rather than allow yourself to be overcome by the demon anger and robbed of your strength, learn to remain calm and confront your feelings with discriminative wisdom. Hold the feeling of anger in your awareness and study how it manifests in your body. Notice how it distorts and directs your thoughts. Make the demon your ally rather than your master.

What you can learn to do with anger you can also learn to do with sadness and depression. Rather than medicate your self with drugs (this includes sex, TV, and other distractions) face and be mindful of the feelings.

Of course it often helps to talk things out with someone who will actually listen to you. In the long run, however, you must often wait upon the unfolding of an inward process. By learning to let go rather than deny your feelings you are in a better position to change their shapes. Your "demons" can thus be transformed into helpers, and energy normally wasted on anger and defensiveness can be used for appropriate action.

The true path to mastery lies not in the magical and the mystical, but in an imaginative combination of inward work and action in the world. This brings us to *Tantra*.

9

Tantra

Tantra may be summed up in the statement: "*nirvana* is *samsara* and *samsara* is *nirvana*."[1] *Nirvana* refers to a condition in which the manufacture of misery has ceased. *Samsara* refers to the round of "birth and death", i.e., your tendency to create misery by *clinging* to the mundane world of transient experience.

The equation of *nirvana* and *samsara* may seem strange if you are used to thinking dualistically. Dualistic thought separates *samsara* from *nirvana* and holds them as opposites.

In the extreme the dualistic position becomes a mysticism that conceives of nirvana as a transcendental state apart from everyday affairs. From such a perspective yoga is perceived as an attempt to attain union with a reality that is entirely *other* than this world of everyday life.

When yoga is interpreted in such mystical terms its practice too often involves world renunciation. Yoga is then viewed as a journey away from the transient, untrustworthy, and "profane" realm of the senses towards the supposed stability and security of some "sacred" absolute.

Tantra rejects such dualism. It views dualistic thinking as a product of the delusion of separation and, therefore, a symptom of ignorance. This rejection of dualism is not a product of philosophic speculation, but arises from the *immediate experience* of yogic concentrative discipline. Tantra holds that when, through practice and desirelessness, the mind becomes truly silent the non-dual nature of things is spontaneously recognized.

When *nirvana* is *samsara* and *samsara* is *nirvana*, the yogic task is no longer construed as one of rejecting the world of the senses in favor of otherworldly mystical experience. Neither is it viewed as one of embracing the profane world and its many pleasures. Embrace and rejection are two sides of another dualism. Either one is a form of entanglement with nature and experience. Instead, tantra advises you to avoid dualistic entanglements by *facing directly whatever your*

---

1.   Bharati, Agehananda. (1975). *The Tantric Tradition.* New York: Samuel Weiser.

present circumstances present and meeting them with practice and desirelessness. This is also the strategy of modern yoga psychology.

According to the tantric approach, the ephemeral world of nature and experience stands before you as a vast playing field on which to exercise your skills of practice and desirelessness. In truth, if you are serious about pursuing yoga or yoga psychology you really have no other choice.

Recall the metaphor of Absolute Reality as seawater with its waves rising and falling. The rising and falling of the waves constitute the relative and transient realm of nature and experience. However ephemeral that realm of relativity may be it is only through the movement of these waves that you experience the Absolute.

Remember that according to this conceptualization the Absolute, as the ground of all experience, cannot itself be experienced. Therefore, there is no experience of the Absolute apart from your experience of transient nature.

The "trick" of tantric yoga is to use the forms of transient nature and experience as vehicles of self-discipline, i.e., means of working on your self without forming attachments. Clearly, this is much easier said that done.

The "danger" of attachment arises not because the sensory world is "profane" or "evil", but simply because its forms are ephemeral. They do not last, but are entirely subject to birth and death. Attachment to these forms can only bring you Misery.

You experience the Absolute only by facing its myriad forms as they actually present themselves to you, not as you would *prefer* them to be presented. Facing them in their actuality creates opportunity. Your present life circumstances are always an opportunity to work on yourself. In other words, your yoga "mat" is wherever you find yourself. Therefore, give up seeking something special and work on yourself now!

In all your present circumstances an important constant is your body. Your body is the principle vehicle of yogic practice. This does not mean that practice is limited to the popular conception of "bodywork". Posture and breath training are an important part of tantric yoga, but hardly its defining aspects. Tantra includes *all* bodily activities and experiences. Your total involvement with life is grist for the tantric mill.

According to tantric tradition the body is a microcosm that mirrors the macrocosm. Since tantra views the universe as a playground for the enjoyment of the "gods", so also is your body. Your body, as a reflection of the cosmos, is a vehicle of enjoyment. Therefore, if you ask, "What is the purpose of life, of being embodied?" the tantric answer is to know Joy.

Tantra views the cosmos as a vast play of creative energy. Traditionally this energy is personified as the goddess, *Shakti*. It is her energy that is the driving power behind all manifestation.

In the Hindu tantric scheme of things *Shakti* is the consort of the god *Shiva*, and their union is the spark of creation. Shiva sows the seed, as it were, and Shakti generates nature and experience. All generativity is seen as a product of *Shakti's* energetic play.

Shiva, however, is known among other things as the god of *destruction*. You might ask then, why is the goddess of generativity hooked up with the god of destruction? This seeming paradox expresses a profound spiritual truth of great importance to yoga.

Ultimately yoga is about letting go. The technical core of yoga, practice and desirelessness, is aimed entirely at your letting go of the sources of misery. In Ignorance you have sought security and constructed what you presume to be a castle of security. The walls of your castle are made of seeking, clinging and defending. They are your prison. *There can be no true creative or generative life while such walls stand!* The walls must be destroyed.

You destroy the walls of your prison by letting go. There is no true creativity without letting go. An artist must let go of past solutions and achievements in order to create anew. If not, then s/he will do little more than grind out the same old stuff. That is not creation; it is repetition. Some might call it "playing safe".

The union of *Shakti* with *Shiva* is at once a moment of destruction and generation. In their moment of sexual climax the separating walls of ego crumble and dualism is let go. In that moment the seed of generation is sown.

In tantric tradition the pathway to letting go is viewed in terms of the body's energy system. This system is conceived as part of your "subtle" body, and comprises a network of *nadis* (energy pathways) and *chakras* (energy centers).

There are many *nadis*, but we need to consider only one, the central channel or *susumna*. This channel is roughly analogous (not identical) to your spinal cord and runs from the perineal region between the anus and the genitals up to the crown of the cerebrum. Along the central channel are arranged seven *chakras*.[2]

According to tantric teaching the energy that operates within this system is the *kundalini-shakti*, i.e., the cosmic *Shakti* as it manifests in the nadis and chakras. Normally, the *kundalini* lies dormant, like a coiled serpent, at the base of the central channel at or near the *muladhara chakra*. The task of the tantric yogi is to

---

2.　Avalon, Arthur. (1974). *The Serpent Power*. Madras: Ganesh & Co.

awaken this serpent energy, force it out of its resting place, and then move it up the central channel to the crown or *sahasrara chakra*.

As *kundalini* courses up the *susumna* it passes through and awakens each of the other six *chakras*. The arrival of *kundalini* at the *sahasrara* is conceived as tantamount to supreme enlightenment. Speaking mythically it is the union of *Shakti* and *Shiva*, the supreme generative moment.

According to tantra, the purpose of existence is enjoyment. However, this enjoyment belongs to *Shiva* (i.e., the Absolute) and not your personal ego. The work of *kundalini* yoga is not one of grasping for an experience, another "spiritual" possession. The awakening at each *chakra* represents a *letting go* of egoic striving. If you can learn both to work and to let go (i.e., cultivate practice and desirelessness) you will increase your capacity for creativity and Joy. If you cannot let go of egoic grasping and experience-mongering, you will turn yoga into a pleasure seeking that leads only to misery.

Egocentric pleasure seeking blocks the flow of Joyous energy in your body. This is because egoism turns everything into competition, comparison, desiring, aversion, and defensive clinging. Defensiveness and clinging constrict the flow of creative energy and Joy.

When you get caught up in seeking and clinging you turn enjoyment into addiction. Addiction begins with pleasure, but eventually descends into pre-occupation with the avoidance of displeasure (e.g., withdrawal). The focus on avoidance results in constricting the flow of your generative energies. You might visualize this as something like a knot tied in a garden hose. Nothing can flow through it.

In the tantric conceptualization this blockage of energy flow is attributed to "knots" or *granthi*. These knots are associated with the *chakras*. That is, the *chakras* are either open to permit a free flow of creative energy or are blocked. According to the tantric scheme the "piercing" of a *chakra* by the rising force of *kundalini* unties or cuts through the resident knot and restores the free flow of your generative energy.

The piercing of the knots and the restoration of energy flow allow *kundalini* to continue its rise up the central channel. According to anecdotal reports the piercing of the knots and the rising of *kundalini* are often accompanied by feelings of heat rising up the spinal cord, bodily shaking and bouncing, hearing buzzing sounds, and seeing flashing lights.

There have been attempts to explain these experiences in neurophysiological, psychodynamic, bioenergetic, and transpersonal psychological terms. The experiential reports have lead to theories about electromagnetic, standing waves in the body, the activation of the vagus nerve, and the orgasm reflex. The *chakras* have been interpreted as symbols of psycho-spiritual development, identified with Freud's erogenous zones, and, as you might suspect, dismissed as new age nonsense.[3]

In my opinion none of the explanations has much relevance for actual practice. The *chakras* were originally described in order to provide the tantric yogi with a set of imaginal supports for meditation. The traditional descriptions of the *chakras* included geometric designs (*yantra*), animals, deities, their consorts, and specific colors to be visualized, as well as *mantra* to be recited. All of these were intended as possible foci for meditative practice. As such they are not symbols of psychic process or spiritual development, but simply tools for meditation.

A tantric practitioner does not visualize an image as a *symbol* of a deity, but as part of a concentrative means to *realize* his or her *essential identity* with the deity. In the non-dual spirit of *samsara* is *nirvana* and *nirvana* is *samsara*, the student's aim is to overcome the delusion of separation from the deity and all creation.

The overcoming of the delusion of separation is the Joyous event traditionally described as the union of *Shakti* and *Shiva*. A usual representation of this event is that of a divine couple locked in a sexual embrace. Many have taken such imagery to signify that tantra is in essence a form of sexual yoga, i.e., that sexual intercourse is a critical part of tantric yogic practice. This conclusion is misleading.

Sex in tantra refers to much more than physical sexual intercourse and its sensual enjoyment. Its primary significance is that of *generativity*. This includes all creative processes from the cosmic and biological to human technical invention and artistic expression. When tantra speaks of freeing your sexual energy it refers to your learning to en-Joy the *full range* of your human creative potential, not just genital pleasure.

Ultimately, the great Joy expressed by the coupling of the cosmic deities is that of liberation from the delusions of separation and freedom from birth and death. In this coupling he becomes her and she becomes him as *nirvana* is *samsara* and *samsara* is *nirvana*.

In medieval India tantric practice fell into one of two branches, the right-handed and left-handed paths. These two paths differed largely in their approaches to what a puritanical Brahmin culture held to be forbidden behaviors. These behaviors were sexual intercourse, eating meat and fish (i.e., animal flesh), eating parched grain, and drinking alcohol. Engaging in any of these was consid-

---

3.   For a review see White, John (Ed.) (1990). *Kundalini: Evolution and Enlightenment.* St. Paul: Paragon.

ered destructive of one's vital energies and thereby detrimental to the practice of yoga. The ejaculation of semen was considered to be particularly wasteful in this regard.

The right-hand practitioners obeyed the proscriptions and did not employ sex, meat, alcohol, etc. in their practices. Sexual symbolism might play a role in imaginal meditative exercises, but actual sexual intercourse was not part of the deal and masturbation was forbidden. The point of their approach was to use *imagination* to awaken *Shakti* within and direct energy accordingly. The union of male and female and the overcoming of dualism were viewed in a purely psycho-spiritual way.

The followers of the left hand path made participation in the forbidden actions a part of their yoga practice and/or worship. Here there actually was a yoga of sexual intercourse, or *lingam-yoni* yoga (*lingam* referring to the male sexual member and *yoni* to the female). Even in this yoga ejaculation was often frowned upon and yogis (i.e., male practitioners, females are called *yoginis*) were trained to retain their semen during the sex act.

Tantric yogis may have induced retrograde ejaculations in an effort to avoid what they feared as a loss of vital energy. In addition, various psychophysiological techniques were used to direct the flow of energy inwardly, i.e., up the central channel to the *sahasrara*.

Whether right or left-handed, the important practice was inward and carried out in a spirit of desirelessness. When actual sexual intercourse was involved it was usually between individuals who had been trained in the appropriate disciplines. Both partners fully appreciated that the sexual exercise involved a conversion of physical pleasure into spiritual Joy through letting go of egoistic grasping and lusting.

The proper tantric attitude is that sex is a natural biological function of the body that is most fully enjoyed when you avoid attachment. Of course, this is true for all natural functions including walking, talking, eating, drinking, and defecating. Aside from its obvious biological importance sex is not special. All bodily functions and actions can be grist for the tantric mill of meditative mindfulness and the cultivation of desirelessness.

Sexual intercourse assumes a "privileged" status because the physical pleasure of orgasm can be very intense. Ideally, this involves sharing Joy with another human being and letting go of egoic boundaries between self and other. More often, however, the intensity of sexual feeling is used as a mere distraction from life's miseries rather than a means of letting go of them. Thus sex becomes one of a host of possible self-medications with a strong potential for addiction.

The problem of sexual addiction seems widespread in our culture. As the poet Gary Snyder has suggested, this may be due to the fact that, for many, sexual intercourse is often the only source of epiphany.[4] Given that sexual intercourse is often confused with love, aggression, and power, you have the perfect karmic circumstances for the ripening of sexual dependency.

Confusions surrounding the meaning of sex have led to a situation in which many people believe that unless they have a "dynamic" sex life they are not truly living or loving. Men and women often equate sex with love and fear that a diminution of sexual activity spells loss of love. If you have sex with your partner four times a week you do not love that person more than if you had sex only twice a month. Sex and love can be a great combination, but they are not the same thing.

According to Freud, all human babies are born "polymorphously perverse". This means that they can experience pleasure from any part of their bodies. Accordingly the infant lives in a state of "erotic unity with all of nature".[5] This condition is akin to the timeless unity of mystical communion.

As a consequence of socialization (i.e., social hypnosis) the capacity to experience pleasure anywhere in the body becomes restricted to specific zones, i.e., oral, anal, and genital. Classical Freudian theory holds the genital focus to represent "maturity", but modern yoga psychology sees the developmental stages as successive constrictions of the natural flow of sexual energy. These constrictions account for the fact that genital sexual excitement is the only source of Joy for so many in our materialist culture.

From this perspective, the piercing of the chakras and the knots represents an undoing of socially imposed constrictions. When *Shakti* finally reaches the crown *chakra* the full flow of sexual energy is again possible and the conversion of pleasure to Joy occurs.

There are two points to consider in all of this. First, the experiences that result from the rising of kundalini are only experiences. They are as transient as any other experience and must not be allowed to become foci of seeking and attachment.

Much of the popular Western literature on tantra overemphasizes and romanticizes the experiential side of yoga. This may make some sense in contrast with purely intellectual treatments, but can leave aspirants with a distorted view of genuine yogic work. It tends to paint yoga, and tantrism in particular, with a sen-

---

4.   This remark appeared in one of Snyder's essays. I regret I cannot supply a reference. I suggest you look in his complete works.

5.   Wilber, Ken. Are the *chakras* real? In White, John (Ed.) (1990). *Kundalini: Evolution and Enlightenment*. St. Paul: Paragon.

sualist brush. An example of this are new age "gurus" who advertise "tantric" yoga as a path to bigger and better orgasms. While technically such claims may have merit, the focus on sensual pleasure turns a by-product of practice into a spiritual detour and even trap. This is why practice must always be paired with the cultivation of desirelessness. Yoga should lead you to freedom rather than addiction.

The second point is that all the talk about *chakras, nadis,* and *granthis* over-complicates the show. Originally described as props for meditation and nothing more, they can be dispensed with entirely. There is no requirement to conceptualize the practice of yoga in these terms. In general it is best to keep things simple.

In the final analysis a *chakra* is a focus of awareness. Visualizing *chakras* is simply one way of helping a student to become aware of his/her own body and the feelings associated with it. Such focusing helps let go of localized holding and tenseness, i.e., unties emotional knots. The result can involve the release of sexual feelings, but emotional and generative freedom is the aim.

The knot of greatest importance is the one that ties you to your body. This is a *knot of delusion* and it doesn't matter where you localize it or if you localize it. It is identification with and dependence upon your body (its actions and experiences) that constricts your Joy with the fear of death. Anything that helps you let go of this knot is all to the good.

So, don't worry about the fact that Hindu yogis may talk about seven *chakras,* Buddhist yogis count only five, and various other systems count them to over 40. All that really matters is that you learn to focus your attention to different areas of your body, become aware of your feelings and tenseness, and then let go. It is the letting go that counts.

Here is how you might look at the rising of *kundalini.* As you move your attention throughout your body, focusing on (and visualizing) each part or area, you try to get a feeling of actually breathing into each part. As you do this try to feel that you are becoming increasingly aware of the feelings and sensations in that area. Then, as you breathe out get a feeling of letting it all go. If you do this in a systematic and complete way you will learn to "breathe away" your body. This weakens the knot of identification with your body.

As you breathe away your body you may notice that a kind of "space" gradually opens. This space becomes a "window" through which memories and associated feelings "rise up" to enter your consciousness. Since the meditative state greatly attenuates the intensity of such feelings the experience will not be traumatic, i.e., you will be able to handle them. The result is more of a joyous release than a trauma revisited.

This is *kundalini* conceived as catharsis and the undoing of defensive holding. Naturally, energy previously tied up in holding is released and made available for natural generative living. As you re-educate yourself to create your life you participate directly in the creation of the cosmos. You ride with the gods and know their Joy. And best of all, it is all perfectly natural.

There is yet another way to look at this. Through meditative self-study (bringing awareness to the body and feelings) you, in effect, face your "demons". In so doing you let go of defensiveness and allow yourself to know the energies that constitute these "demons". They are, after all, the creatures of your own fear and defending. As repression is relaxed these "demonic" energies are transformed into spontaneous naturalness and benevolent generativity. This is how *samsara* becomes *nirvana*.

Therefore, greet each situation you face with practice and desirelessness. Pay attention to what is! The present situation is all you ever have and all you ever really need if you remain awake and aware.

The true unity of all opposites is recognized when you see through the delusion of separation. If you happen to be having sex, well, great. "En-joy" it. If you are walking in the woods, paddling a canoe, feeding a baby, adding a column of figures, sipping green tea, trying to sell an automobile, or sitting on the toilet, *be all there* and enjoy. If something gets in the way of your enjoyment, take appropriate external and/or internal action! Above all, do not cling to any of it, but keep letting go! You can always let go a little bit more.

10

Final Thoughts

If this were a lecture rather than a book I would now ask for your questions. Since we are not face-to-face I must *assume* what your questions are based on my experience with students in the past.

This section will necessarily involve some repetition. I do not apologize for that. Anything worth saying once should be worth saying twice or more.

Never forget that yoga psychology is rooted in *practice*, the yogic practice of cultivating mental stillness through concentration. Even though I may call upon modern psychological ideas from time to time the prime root remains classical yoga.

Always keep in mind that practice and philosophy are not the same. Philosophy is verbal and conceptual, a search by the intellect to solve problems posed by the intellect. Most of these problems exist because of the intellect. They are the products of thought and rooted in thinking. As such they cannot be put to rest by thought.

Don't misunderstand me. Philosophical issues do *reflect* certain deep human concerns: What is real? How do I find happiness? How should I conduct my life? What happens when I die? Intellect cannot answer these questions. When intellect tackles such issues it only complicates the mental world. Intellect can make a helpful approach to concrete problems in the outer world, e.g., how to build a better computer, design cleaner automobile engines, make waterproof fabric, etc. Intellect cannot cope satisfactorily with spiritual, existential, or relationship problems because these are largely *internal* and subjective.

Yoga psychology addresses human dilemmas through discipline, the discipline of *stilling* rather than exercising mental process. It first recognizes the presence of human misery and then guides you to a way to free yourself of it by looking within for its roots. Further, yoga psychology argues that to free yourself of Misery, you must act. Action is the only way to turn from the virtual world of concepts, fancy, and unending internal conversation to the realm of the actual. Since yoga psychology looks to your inward life it leads to acting upon yourself, within.

The yogic call to act within and work on yourself reflects its assertion that you cannot rely on some "other" or "higher" power to deliver you from misery. You must do the work yourself. Yoga psychology is *self*-discipline and not a form of worship.

The charge to work on your self does not go over well these days. Many object that work and effort are not necessary because Truth is already here and now, etc. I once met a "spiritual teacher" who had convinced himself that "everything is perfect just as it is." According to him all one had to do was just "be" and "go with the flow".

I agree that the Truth is already here and now, but you must then ask why you still suffer miseries. Yoga psychology teaches that you suffer life's miseries because you have learned *habits* of misery. Habits, call them "bad" *karma* if you want, generate an obscuring veil of mental complications that blind you to "what is". *If you want to remove that veil you must practice some kind of mental discipline.* Habits of mental complication can only be removed by habits of mental quiet.

Removing old habits calls for effort. "Effort" is a bad word in many circles. There are always those who, dominated by inertia, seek to remain comfortable by not moving. They worship the bird in the hand and have no interest in the birds in the bush. Yoga psychology asks you to let go of the bird in hand and go for the birds in the bush. When you get it, let it go as well.

Importers of the wisdom of the East also speak of the Dao and how "non-striving" is the answer. It is true that there is a doctrine of "action through in-action". Of course these are only words. True *practitioners* of the Dao, like those of Zen Buddhism, often advise students to take up one of the arts, e.g., *taijiquan*, calligraphy, etc. These all require practice. Those who take up *taijiquan* (some call it a Chinese yoga) soon discover that they have lots of habits that need changing. They need to learn all over again how to stand, how to walk, how to push and twist.

A Taijiquan teacher once said to me, "You practice Taiji for five to ten years and then you begin to learn Taiji. After another five to ten years of learning maybe you can forget Taiji and just flow." Too many today want to jump in and start flowing without first practicing. They want the supposed goal, but cannot bring themselves to take on the ten to twenty years of work. It is the same with yoga and yoga psychology.

In a very real sense there is no goal. If you cultivate desirelessness along with practice you will not be concerned with any goal. Similarly there are no "arrived" or "perfect masters". There are only those who learn how to work on themselves with the understanding that there will always be something to work on. There is no end to practice for practice is its own end.

Some object that meditation is a waste because no amount of meditation will bring Being into being. They point out that Being already is! Of course Being already is. It is equally true, however, that if your spiritual eyes are closed in the sleep of ignorance, you must awaken and open them in order to see!

What if someone has glued your eyelids shut? This is not a whimsical comment, but a metaphor for the miseducation to which most have been exposed. If you have been mis-educated through physical, psychological, or spiritual abuse then you have most likely been hypnotized to a life of delusion. Shall you simply "let it be"? Do you wish to remain in such a trance state?

The Buddha's first noble truth asks that we all face the fact that life comes with a full share of frustration, dissatisfaction, and anxiety. Buddha was no chirpy cheerleader who refused to face the truth of things. Following the age old dictates of yoga he left the comforts of his habitual palace life to face the truths of old age, sickness, and death. He went within and by so doing awakened to Truth!

Some present yoga as religion. This is very common since many teachers come from India where devotional forms of yoga predominate and the line between religion and yoga is blurred. Nonetheless, yoga and yoga psychology are not religion. The greatest psychological treatise of yoga, the *Yogasutra of Patanjali*, was conceptually rooted in *Sankhya*, an *atheistic* philosophy.

It is true that Patanjali's *Yogasutra* teaches that concentration on an image of a deity is *one* way to achieve concentration. Other supports might serve as well, however. In yoga the image of the deity is used to intensify concentration and ultimately quiet the mind. The aim is *mental silence*. In religion the practice of concentration is normally used to intensify devotion. In that case worship of the deity takes precedence over quieting the mind. The religious approach can thus pose an impediment to the completion of the yogic path. As long as the image of a deity is present there is no mental silence and the ultimate aim of yoga is postponed.

There is another issue of importance here, however, that of letting go or "surrender". When devotion to a deity is used in yoga it is a psychological ploy to help the student let go. For many, letting go is more easily understood when put in terms of surrender to a deity or some "higher power". Yoga psychology may use such an approach when suitable as a means of undermining egoism. Eventually, however, the student must let go of the image and idea of the deity. The end point of yogic concentration is absorption *without* an object, i.e., complete mental silence. Once there is silence the true nature of the self and the deity become clear.

Is the attainment of complete mental silence a real possibility? Perhaps it is, perhaps it is not. I have heard some say that complete silence is simply inconceivable. They argue that as *karma* forces bodies to act it also forces minds to think. In the end you must find out for yourself through practice. Yoga does teach that concentration without an object is the eventual goal of concentration.

Here are some principles from practice. You cannot think thought away. That is, no amount of mental effort will silence the mind because mental effort is mental noise. You can learn to concentrate on one object, however, and you can use that concentration to take your mind back to its source. Even though such concentration is not silence it is, theoretically, the place from which you can jump into silence.

The jump occurs when you *let go* of mind. The silence is one that has always been there in the background and the spaces between your thoughts. Silence is not created by concentration, but is the ever-present ground of all mental process. When mental process becomes calm this silence begins to reveals itself. Don't take my word for it; test it for yourself.

Existentially speaking, you must come to a point via one-pointed concentration where you can drop into the silence without any thought of something to land on or someone to catch you. This plunge into silence or emptiness is the ultimate leap of faith into absorption without an object. This is not a faith *in* something, but an *inward willingness to let go* completely.

You may call this "surrender" if you want to, but it is not surrender *to* something. The movement from absorption with an object to absorption without an object is a true "leap of faith". Not that leap in which reason capitulates to belief, but a willingness to fall into the "void". Ultimately, *this is a total acceptance of personal death.*

For the vast majority, religion and other spiritual pursuits function as a way of denying or escaping death. It begins with a fear of death (the final source of affliction to emerge from Ignorance) and ends with a mythology of transcendence, resurrection, reincarnation of the individual, or some such deliverance. These mythologies present images of the escape and avoidance of real death. Yoga on the other hand asks you to face your death squarely, and argues that only by facing death can you hope to understand what it is and what it isn't. That is, you must accept the inevitability of your bodily death and allow yourself to become familiar with it.

The path of familiarity with death is meditation, the silencing and/or letting go of all mental process. In that process the question becomes not how to transcend death, but to discover who is this "I" that dies.

This is the essential yogic project of reversing the emergence of your mind, of turning your mind back upon itself. By taking your mind back to its source, the source of the "I"-thought, you root out the fear of death and all other sources of affliction that cause misery. This includes, of course, seeing through the delusion of separation. The mind that has been returned to its source lets go of the sources of affliction and finds itself rooted in a profound silence; a silence that is the ground not only of mind, but all appropriate and effective action.

Do not think that reversing the process of mental emergence is some kind of developmental regression. From the yogic perspective the important emergence is not a historical process of chronological growth, but one that occurs all the time from moment to moment. The best way to understand this is to become a detached observer of your own mental process and begin to discern what transpires from moment to moment. The best way to do this is through the practice of one-pointed concentration.

When you practice concentration you inevitably become an observer of your mental process. This happens, by the way, even if it is not your intent. In fact, when you practice concentration making such observations should not be your intent for that would interfere with the concentration. Concentration should involve only the one point with no idea of any goal whatsoever.

In recent years some psychologists interested in Eastern spiritual paths have suggested that meditative disciplines offer ways to study mental process. They appear to suggest that meditation represents a kind of spiritual "technology" that could be put to work in the interests of science, e.g., cataloging altered states of consciousness.

Such projects may indeed be served by interviewing experienced practitioners. I think, however, it is an error to conceive of meditative techniques as the "psychic" analogs of EEG, MRI, and other Western investigative technologies. The Western technologies represent extensions and amplifications of the human senses and are conceived as tools of objective study. The amplified senses reach *outward* toward objects. This is true even if the object is beneath the skin, e.g., the activities of cerebral neurons.

In yoga, concentration is not used for objective study, but for *subjective realization*. The aim is to learn to *let go* of attachment to mental process and all that goes with it. When you concentrate on one object you let go of all other objects. Having let go of all other objects you are *fully present* to the selected object.

The project of letting go is different from that of natural science and may even be antithetical to it. Natural science strives to *accumulate* knowledge. There is little in its discipline that is designed to counter egocentric attachment to these accumulations. On the contrary, it has been my experience that students are encouraged to get caught up in *competition* to publish or perish, etc. Scientists can get very nasty with one another when such competition rears its head.

Scientists are also concerned with the utility of their findings. This is as it should be since science is clearly involved with understanding the workings of nature for the material betterment of humanity. Yoga is largely indifferent to material betterment. Its concern is with spiritual awakening and letting go, not with the accumulation of material benefits.

Yogic concentration has been portrayed by some psychologists as unnatural or forced.[1] Such criticism has contrasted concentrative meditation with Buddhist mindfulness meditation, a technique portrayed as open, flowing, and "fully present" to the "here and now".

My own exposure to mindfulness techniques reveals that they usually begin with *concentration* on a single point, e.g., the rhythm of breathing or the movement of one's feet when walking slowly and deliberately. None of the Eastern teachers whose workshops I have attended have ever suggested that beginning meditators should simply "go with the flow".

Within the classical yogic tradition concentrative meditation eventually leads to absorption without an object, a condition that can be readily described as one of being "fully present to the here and now". In brief, my personal experience does not support a hard and fast distinction between concentration and mindfulness. Once you get past conceptualizing I doubt if there is any real difference. In the end, you must practice and see for yourself.

I have said relatively little about reincarnation. This is because, contrary to popular understanding, yoga (and therefore yoga psychology) doesn't teach reincarnation. While a great many Eastern people believe in some kind of personal reincarnation it is not a part of classical yogic teaching. I was taught, for example, that no true student of yoga would have any interest in such reincarnation since it would represent further turnings on the painful rack of mundane existence. In other words, if personal reincarnation were to exist, it should be avoided at all costs.

---

1.   The Gestalt psychologist Fritz Perls was representative of this view.

As for modern yoga psychology, it understands the individual personality to be an entirely fanciful construction of mental process having no status as an entity. Given such a view, the idea of any kind of personal reincarnation makes no sense whatever. This is not to say that our actions have no consequences or that those consequences do not extend beyond the time frame of our individual lives.

When karma is taken into consideration there is a sense in which a kind of "rebirth" does indeed take place. This is not the rebirth of any "little old me", however. Reincarnation makes the most sense when you consider individuals as *embodiments* of certain human traits or characteristics. For example, compassion, benevolence, and other powerful dispositions are embodied again and again in the world. The present Dalai Lama is said to be the reincarnation of *Avalokitesh-vara* (*Chenrezig* in Tibetan), the *bodhisattva* of infinite compassion. There is no question in my own mind that he is a present manifestation of that spirit. To the extent that his life succeeds in awakening compassion in others you could say that compassion truly transmigrated from one body to another.

Nonetheless, yoga psychology asserts without qualm that your individual, ego-centric personality will not survive your bodily death. There is really nothing personal that survives other than the effects of your actions.[2] The popular understanding of reincarnation, like the popular view of heaven, is a fancy born of the need to deny personal death. Yoga psychology teaches that rather than deny death you must face your fear of it and seek the courage to leap off the cliff into emptiness. Do not cling. Do not grasp. If you find this discomfiting you have work to do on yourself.

I have referred to both yoga and yoga psychology as "psycho-spiritual" disciplines. "Spiritual" is a word that is used so widely as to have nearly lost all meaning. To me yoga psychology is "spiritual" in the sense that it asks you to *examine your internal life* and face the issues of personal identity, death, and the making and unmaking of Misery. All of these, however, boil down to the question of *identity*. What is the point of examining the nature of your death or your miseries if you do not know who "you" are? Here is a "*mantram*" for you:

Spiritual awakening is the realization that

You *can* be your self.

To be your Self you must first *find* your Self.

To find your self is to lose all Misery.

---

2.   Some will object that this view is not consistent with the *Sankhya* concept of *Purusha* as expressed in the *Yogasutra*. They are correct in this. The view expressed in the chapter is closer to non-dual *Vedanta*, and may be even closer to early Buddhism.

There is nothing esoteric or occult in this. Nothing is "hidden" from you other than those things you fear to face. There is no "special" knowledge other than knowing your True Self-nature.

This means that you can truly *be* your Self instead of being a hypnotized and sleepwalking creature of social conditioning and manipulation. There is no need to let others define who you are. If you would truly know your self you have only to look within. Of course, this inward turn will be against the grain of years of psychological habit.

To find and know yourself requires that you *work on yourself* to *undo* the habits of Ignorance, Egoism, Desire, Aversion, and Clinging. Please note the word "undo". All yogic work is aimed at undoing the Ignorance that occludes your self-recognition. In this respect there is nothing to gain from practicing yoga psychology; you have only to lose your misery.

Undoing the machinery of misery is a tall order. It asks you to embark on a course of self-study and not rest until you have learned to discern the false from the true and recognized the *source of your own mind*. This requires that you cultivate mental stillness by letting go of mental noise.

Does yoga teach that all mental process is nothing but noise? Yes and no. Much of your mental activity is useful in coping with daily life and that includes the project of realizing your creaturely potential. You do need to know how to best use your mental faculties to solve problems and live creatively. You cannot do this, however, while Ignorance rules your mind. To diminish the influence of Ignorance you must quiet your mind. Ignorance and its spawn (Egoism, Desire, Aversion, and Clinging to Life) cannot operate without mental process. *When your mind is quiet Ignorance loses its grip and you can recognize Truth.*

When you begin to understand the role your own mind plays in doing the work of Ignorance it may be tempting to take up arms against it. Do not do this! Your mind is not your enemy. Ignorance is your enemy. It is not mind in general that causes Misery, but mind in the grip of Ignorance.

The followers of Sun Myung Moon (i.e., the "Moonies") were fond of saying, "thinking is stinking". They were wrong. What stinks is not thinking, i.e., mental process, but the inability to discern truth from falsehood and reality from unreality. You are urged to practice mental quiet not because mental process "stinks", but because it is so easily co-opted by Ignorance. When Ignorance has been rooted out, you can use mental process in those areas to which it is suited.

Sometimes I speak of mental "silence" and at other times mental "steadiness". A mind that is steady stays "on point", i.e., it is concentrated on or absorbed by its object. A steady mind is not fickle, distracted, or sluggish. A steady mind is one-pointed and free of conflict.

A steady mind permits action that is sure, smooth, and spontaneously appropriate to its circumstances. A steady mind does not worry about success and failure, winning and losing. A steady mind is uncomplicated and calm. A silent mind, on the other hand, is one that has let go of all objects and no longer clings. This is absorption without an object. Mind and body have dropped away.

Now, can you drop dropping? If you can you are left with spontaneous naturalness in all things. True dexterity in action manifests without your knowing it. (If you miss the opportunity for praise and congratulations here you are back on the karmic rack!)

Some preach that once you quiet your mind and experience "great emptiness" you are truly "saved". That is nonsense. First of all, there is nothing "great" about emptiness. Emptiness is empty, no greatness, no reward, no praise, no diploma. Second, as long as there is a "you" and any thought of "salvation" you are not saved. Forget about salvation and you have a chance. The same goes for "enlightenment". Don't seek; just stay awake.

Does "spontaneous naturalness" mean that you become really good at everything? No. It means that you are not awkward and anxious over concern for success v. failure, praise v. blame, etc. To be good at something you have to practice the relevant skills and apply them with concentration. Skills are important in coping with everyday life, and you need them in order to realize your potential. It is important, therefore, that you discover what you need to learn and find someone to teach you. Then you must practice! The great "trick" in all this is to apply skills without becoming entangled in competition and comparison. It may be difficult to apply effort without invoking ego, but it can be done. In sum, concentration promotes spontaneous naturalness by bracketing out distractions and allowing well-practiced skills to manifest.

You may have been confused by the discussion of the relationship of absolute reality to both actual and virtual reality. A review may help. It is important to know that all of these terms refer to *conceptual* distinctions. "Absolute", "relative", "actual", and "virtual" are all concepts, i.e., mental constructions used to classify types of knowledge and experience. They provide a kind of "map" that you can use in navigating through your own mental processes. If you do not find this map useful, let it go.

The domain of "actuality" refers to knowledge rooted in immediate sensory experience as opposed to conceptual knowledge mediated by words. Although knowledge gained through testimony involves verbal communication it, theoretically, reflects another person's immediate, non-verbal sensory experience. That is, an "actual" object is assumed to have initiated the process.

"Fancy" refers to knowledge that arises from words alone. Fancies are "pure" verbalisms, i.e., the relevant mental images or objects are not evoked by immediate sensory activity, but by words. Conceptualization is the most common form of fancy, and may even represent the majority of your mental processes.

The distinction between actuality and fancy is not always clear. This is because much right and wrong knowledge comes from testimony and therefore involves words. First of all, sensory experience is probably never "pure". Psychological studies have shown that it is very difficult to separate sensation from cognition. For example, our experience of colors is greatly influenced by the color names we have learned. Non-verbal expectations also "flavor" what appears to our senses.

Once words enter the picture a lot can happen. Who can say that someone's testimonial words do not also evoke fancies? I suspect that most misunderstandings occur because one speaker's words evoke images in the mind of a listener that turn out to be inconsistent with the images the speaker had in mind. They may be using the same words, but still not be on the same "page".

It would be a mistake to assume that the use and effects of fancy are always obvious. Most likely the opposite is the case. In the context of both external and internal conversations we repeatedly evoke fancy without realizing it, and as a result images of right and wrong knowledge get mixed with fancy in a way that makes discernment difficult. It becomes very easy to lose sight of which images are fancies and which are not, and as a result we easily confuse actual with virtual realities. Advertisers, politicians, and other specialists in hypnotic sloganeering take great advantage of this.

Perhaps it is best to think of your experience as a mix of actual and virtual images in which the balance between the two is constantly shifting. If the mix is dominated by immediate sensory input it is more actual that virtual. A mix dominated by fancy, however, pushes things toward the virtual. The cultivation of a concentrated presence of mind is needed to enable discrimination between the actual and the virtual, and to gain sufficient detachment to control the balance.

While the distinction between actual and virtual perceptions can be difficult, one thing is very clear. Both worlds of actuality and fancy are products of your mental processes and belong to the ephemeral realm of nature and experience. As such they are transient and cannot be depended upon as a source of security.

Why do I insist on harping on this? In the face of an insecure world of constant change you become anxious and seek security, something to hold onto. The typical response is a retreat into fancy and the construction of virtual realities that give an appearance of stability and security. Such responses may function as a temporary "opiate", but they will fail unless they lead you to face Truth. Know that the path to Truth is one that leads you to "see through" both actuality and virtuality, and especially that it is not something dished out by some ecclesiastic, academic, or political authority. Real Truth must arise from within you.

What is the role of the "absolute" in all of this? The term "absolute" refers to a reality conceived as permanent and independent, a reality not subject to the changes of nature and experience. The conceptualization of an absolute represents an intellectual attempt to compensate for the realization that there is nothing permanent and reliable in nature and experience. For millennia human beings have looked around themselves, seen nothing but the continuing changes of nature and experience, and asked, "what in all of this can we find to rely upon?"

The absolute is usually conceived as some kind of "higher" or transcendental power, a deity or cosmic force, etc. Given an overwhelming human tendency to personify, the absolute is almost always framed as a god or goddess with some degree of human form and/or motivation. Even when a religion preaches that God cannot be portrayed in any way we still hear that God is "angry", "loving", "jealous", "has a plan for us", etc. Very few are comfortable with the absolute as an abstraction.

I once looked up "god" in the *Dictionary of Philosophy and Religion: Eastern and Western Thought* by William L. Reese.[3] That work gives 64 conceptualizations that have been constructed by theologians and philosophers over the centuries. This gives testimony to the difficulties involved in seeking a purely conceptual solution to the problem.

Reality, Truth, the Absolute, cannot be encompassed by any image or conceptualization. There is nothing in either actual or virtual reality that you can point to and say, truthfully, "That is absolute," or "This is the absolute!" All yoga psychology is willing to say about the Absolute is that it is Pure Being.

If you must have more I offer the following conceptualization: There are actually five ways to view the relationship of Being to the forms of nature and experience depending on how you place your attention. Reverting to the metaphor of the sea and its myriad waves, these ways can be described as follows:

1. You behold the totality of the Great Sea of Being.
2. Your attention shifts to individual forms *as they emerge* from the sea.

---

3.   Humanities Press, Atlantic Highlands, N.J., 1980.

3. Attention then narrows to the individual forms and you lose sight of the sea.

4. You then see each individual form as composed, essentially, of seawater.

5. You leap in and start swimming.

The fifth position is not a "point of view", but represents letting go of all views to bathe in unpremeditated naturalness.

"Leaping in" includes commitment to practice and letting go of all dualisms. There is no contradiction in this. You might think that practice implies dualism, i.e., a seeker and something sought. Such a construction does not do justice to practice, however. Practice really has no separate goal. In yoga psychology practice is its own goal. It is known as *practice with desirelessness*!

Dualism originates with the feeling of separation and becomes conceptualized with the aid of language. Language allows the primal dualism of self and other to multiply into an apparent universe of dualities. These disappear when you silence your mental process.

Practice enables you to become more fully aware of your immediate sensory world, the world of the actual. As one-pointed concentration becomes concentration without an object there develops a felt sense of "open space". This "open space" is not an object of experience, however; so don't fall into the trap of looking for it.

Some might say that the sense of open space involves a "glimpse" of the ground of pure awareness and/or Being. This goes too far, I think, in suggesting an experiential goal. Goals support seeking, and seeking is inherently egoistic. Remember, there can be no experience of the ground of experience.

There may be those who take the concept of "openness" as an invitation to embrace anything and everything that comes along. This also is a mistake. In openness there is neither embrace nor rejection. It certainly does not mean the indiscriminate embrace of everything in your path.

For example, some teachers present "openness" as indulging in sex and other desire-driven behavior any time one feels inclined. They tell their followers "do what feels good". I have even heard of "gurus" who preach sexual intercourse as a tantric imperative and goad workshop attendees to let go of their inhibitions and dance around without their clothes on. There may be something useful in dancing nude in the moonlight, but I am not sure what it is. There is no question, however, that indiscriminate sex can spread disease and cause both physical and psychological harm. A true student of yoga avoids behavior that might be harmful to self or others.

As for "getting naked" there is no requirement in yoga or yoga psychology that you either undress in public or practice without clothes. This is not medieval India where naked *sadhus* are part of the landscape. In any event "nakedness" is a metaphor for having let go of dependence on things that are not dependable. Since nothing in nature and experience is ultimately dependable, yoga psychology does ask you to learn to go "naked" into the world. To do otherwise invites misery.

You do need to become aware of and let go of your *unconscious* inhibitions. This does not mean that you should scuttle the practice of ethical restraints and observances. Ethical training rules are an important part of yogic discipline.

Restraints, for example, should be exercised with *fully conscious* understanding and intent. That is, you should know what you are doing when you do it and why. This is very different from neurotic avoidance motivated by anxiety. Yogic restraint must not be confused with the injunctions imposed by repressive miseducation.

Observances may be misinterpreted as well as restraints. A good example is the Mahayana Buddhist emphasis on compassion. There sometimes seems to be an atmosphere in Buddhist *sanghas* that being compassionate is a commandment, i.e., if you are a Buddhist you *should* be compassionate and shame on you if you are not. No one actually says this out loud, but if you show me a *sangha*, ashram, monastery, or convent, I will find you examples of such self-righteousness.

Do not misunderstand me. True compassion is a wondrous thing. Ideally, compassion blossoms forth as the result of the weakening of egocentrism and the recognition that the separation of self and other is a delusion. Like love, compassion is a spontaneous consequence of the dissolving of the sense of separation and disconnection. It cannot be commanded.

I am aware that Tibetan Buddhist practice includes techniques intended to foster compassion. One example is *tonglen*, a practice in which one imagines breathing in another person's suffering, reducing it to a "black seed" in the heart, transmuting that seed into one of joy and blessings, and then exhaling these in a powerful stream toward the sufferer. From the standpoint of yoga psychology, such a technique of practicing compassion toward those who suffer comes under the heading of the *practice of contraries* discussed in Chapter VII.

Yoga psychology does not regard these as magical practices, but as inward psychological disciplines to alter one's own attitudes toward those in misery. They are not so much compassion "on" switches as ways of weakening egocentric avoidance of those who are in pain. They are most effective when carried out in the context of your own work on yourself.

All of this talk of "working on your self" may sound self-centered, but it is not. It is in the spirit of the following famous bits of advice: "Charity (*caritas*) begins at home," "To thine own self be true, thou canst not then be false to any man," and "Love thy neighbor as thyself". The last implies that if you truly love yourself you will also love your neighbor because *you are not separate*!

All this means is that the road to compassion is paved with practice. If you cultivate mental steadiness, silence, and desirelessness you will eventually come to the recognition of Truth that releases genuine compassion.

Given the importance of practice and the need for a teacher to guide that practice, it is time to discuss how you find a teacher. There are a number of things to consider. First, if all you want is a good class for postures check out the Yellow Pages, the bulletin boards at local book stores, or the message boards at natural foods markets and restaurants. *The Yoga Journal* publishes an annual directory of teachers that may be a useful source of information. Don't forget to ask friends.

It is wise to shop around. Visit classes and take a trial class if it is permitted. If such a trial is not allowed it probably isn't the place for you anyway. By all means talk to students who have been taking the class and see what they say. Ask if there have ever been any problems, e.g., harsh criticism, fostering of competition, favoritism, sexual predation, etc. If you want to be thorough you might locate people who dropped out of a class and question them.

There are many good reasons for dropping or not taking a class. Posture training is offered in a wide variety of styles and some may be more suitable for you than others. Styles can range from near aerobic to more quiet and gentle approaches. There are several kinds of "power" yoga that emphasize strength and endurance. There is even one school that conducts classes with the room temperature around 100 degrees Fahrenheit. Many of these style variations reflect marketing strategies rather than actual yogic method. My bias would steer you away from the aerobic or power types, but you must make up your own mind. Some of the more gentle approaches can go to the other extreme and fail to offer any real challenge.

My own bias is to avoid any teacher who comes on like a drill instructor or otherwise appears to try to fit all students into one tight little mold. I also think small classes are usually better than large ones. You need a class where you can get some individual attention. To my way of thinking there is no point in attending a huge class where you never get to work directly with the teacher.

With some classes you may be asked to sign a contract for a certain number of sessions. Now you are in potential rip-off territory. Read any such contract very carefully (large and small print) and know that, fair or not, your teacher may be more interested in running a business than in nurturing your spiritual freedom.

Avoid any class in which the teacher or the students foster competition. It is hard enough to avoid competition and comparison within your own mind without its being encouraged by the teacher. I would be very suspicious of any class that employed a system of rankings. Such systems may have a place in the martial arts, but even this is doubtful. I recall a student of mine who had studied karate. She told me her sensei once described the black belt as a white one that had simply become dirty with practice. Then there is the remark by Mr. Miyagi, played by Pat Morita in the film *The Karate Kid*. When his young student asked him what kind of belt he had, he replied something like, "Sears and Roebuck, $9.95."

Forget ranks and competition. You are to take a class in order to learn to work on your self, and this has absolutely nothing to do with how "advanced" you or other students may be. I know of far too many students who can *perform* very photogenic postures, but haven't the foggiest idea how to use them to work on themselves. Posture work in yoga is really part of an *inward* discipline rather than outward display.

Your greatest challenge in this day and age will be to find a posture class that offers any real spiritual work. Some teachers will make a stab at teaching meditation techniques, but the majority will offer little more than lip service and clichés. This doesn't mean that the posture work isn't any good, but it may mean that you will need to look elsewhere for genuine spiritual guidance.

You may be able to find a spiritual group that offers some posture work. This is more likely in a large metropolitan area or perhaps a college or university town. In seeking a spiritual group you should apply the same cautions as advised for posture classes. Be aware that competition and comparison may be harder to spot in these groups, but they will be there. Such things are very hard to eliminate since we all bring them with us.

In any kind of group be on the look out for teacher favoritism or "senior" students who are not adequately supervised. Look within yourself and ask if you feel inwardly supported. Do you feel terrified at the thought of making some kind of breach of local etiquette or procedure? If you do, find someone you feel you can trust (ideally the teacher) and discuss the problem. You may be projecting something and could use some reassurances.

Fear of failure may not be all pure projection, however. Groups founded by teachers from the East, e.g., India, Tibet, Japan, etc., whose core teaching may be spiritually fine, often come wrapped in cultural customs that have no relevance to actual spiritual work. Much depends on how rigidly customs are followed and how "transgressions" are handled. I know of a man who joined a Zen group and initially had a terrible time with the "samurai" culture in that he was often fearful of making a "mistake". He stuck with it, however, and eventually the cultural irrelevancies blended into the background and no longer interfered with his practice. He learned to let them go. If such a climate can teach you flexibility it may be all to the good. If you simply conform and become another robot in a robe it is not so good.

Beware of self-righteousness, theirs and yours. Spiritual groups tend to be hothouses of self-righteousness. A good teacher will be sensitive to this and raise the issue when necessary. In this regard it is best that you look to your own issues and not get entangled in judging others. Work on yourself and avoid trying to "work on" someone else. As you work on yourself compassion will grow and you will find yourself capable of being supportive and genuinely helpful. Don't force it. Be honest with yourself.

There may be some advantages to taking on foreign customs as long as they are not egocentric affectations. Having to learn different customs may help you shake up old habits as your attention is awakened from automaticity. For example, coping with meal service at a Zen retreat can be like learning Taijiquan; it becomes an opportunity to practice concentration in the context of movement. All this can be helpful as long as you can avoid joining the robots.

Some spiritual groups have so many students or devotees that contacts with the teacher are very limited. Too often all you can get is a 30-second glance or touch once or twice a year when the "guru" is in town. Depending upon your expectations and beliefs these brief moments can mean a great deal. My personal bias, however, is that if you are to be properly guided you need much more personal contact than that. Ideally you need opportunities for one-on-one instruction. Groups that do not offer such opportunities may have little to offer beyond worshipful subservience.

Ideally, you need a teacher who can know you well enough to assess your spiritual condition. Such a teacher must be able to hold the mirror before you and help you confront your inner demons. Yoga psychology is not in the business of passing out spiritual candy, and it is never enough to merely sit and listen to sermons on "sweetness and light". You need to be given real food, even if it is sometimes very hard to chew.

Modern public relations people tend to portray spiritual teachers as serene saints or gentle, laughing Buddhas, free of all anxiety and care. Teachers, however, are quite human and come in many shapes and sizes. They may manifest themselves in a variety of ways depending on a student's needs and their own personalities (which they do have).

A real teacher will not shrink from pointing out your demons. After all becoming aware of them is the first step in letting them go. How a teacher does this will depend, in part, on how open or closed you are to the mirroring of your spiritual condition. Some students require gentleness while others need to be dealt with more vigorously. I often needed a little "shaking up" before I saw the point.

You may think at times that your teacher is anything but a sweet and saintly person as you feel yourself being pushed faster than you want to go. I am not speaking about posture work so much as psychological re-education. Do you remember the story of the tiger cub that gagged on his first bite of meat? He was pushed to go against his habits. This is where trust in your teacher comes in. You need to be able to trust that s/he is working with your best interests in mind and not just getting off on being a self-styled "crazy guru". It may not always be comfortable because yoga psychology is not an ego trip and comfort is not the aim. More often than not what you call "comfort" is an egocentric delusion that prevents you from facing your fears and doing what you need to do.

Know, however, that a good teacher will not give you a challenge you cannot meet. The challenge may stretch you, but it will not break you. Your teacher should be perceptive *enough* to detect what you can and what you cannot handle. S/he will not take your crutches away without first helping you become strong enough to stand without them. Of course, if you have come to love your crutches you may not fully appreciate what is taking place.

Trust in your teacher is not all you need. You also need faith in your Self. You need the faith that will enable you to leap off the precipice into the void. I am not trying to be dramatic here. The void is always directly in front of you waiting in the very next moment. Any time you are moved out of your comfort and habits to do something new you leap into the void.

A word of caution may be in order here. There is no virtue in doing "new" things just for the sake of novelty and never just to *prove* something. I know people who think that it is spiritual to take up bungee jumping, hang-gliding, and the like. They talk a great deal about "going to the edge" and facing their fears, etc. There may be something to this, but too often such people overlook other "edges" that are always there as a part of ordinary living. For example, one of the most difficult things I have ever done was to express disapproval at a joke that contained an ethnic slur. I don't like social rejection any more than the next person, and raining on someone's bigotry parade could easily lead to it. I do think, however, that we all have a responsibility to show our rejection of such "humor". This can be done with a minimum of rancor, but there is still risk involved. You will never see me bungee jumping, but I do hope you will not find me "chickening out" when bigotry raises its head.

You should know that not all teachers are designated as such. Often the "world in general" moves in with lessons to be learned. Life is full of such challenges, e.g., illness, injury, flat tires and other equipment breakdowns, or the homeless "bum" that looms before you asking for "help". What do you do? How do you respond? What is the right thing to do? Are "right" and "wrong" useful constructs? What is true "help" anyway? Oops! Too late! The moment has passed. Never fear, however, another "test" is around the corner so stay awake!

Also, consider this; any time you adopt a preference you create opposition and conflict. Desire always leads to Aversion. Aversion produces defensiveness and invites repression. Since you want to think well of yourself you must reject all that you judge to be "ill" within yourself. If you collect guilty secrets you will waste energy hiding them. Your shadow will grow so long it becomes a shackle.

No one enjoys being confronted with his or her own "shadow". Ugly and fearsome things lurk there, e.g., guilty secrets, personal demons, and the ever lurking sense of separation. The exposure of your shadow is necessary, however, if you are to free yourself from Misery. You need not parade it before others; becoming a "therapy show-off" is a dodge. You do need to face it yourself. Defending your self against exposure only serves Egoism and represents Aversion. Undoing egoism requires letting go of defenses and with them the fear of exposing what they defend. This is the real meaning of "going naked" into the world.

The yogic literature contains legends of great yogis who confronted and tamed demons. The demons were converted to forces, even deities, which aided the yogis' spiritual efforts. You must do the same. All "demonic" forces represent energy not at your disposal. Through practice you can learn to let go of defensiveness and free that energy for constructive effort. This is how demons become your helpers. So, do not fear your demons, face them, learn their names, and command them.

Remember that Ignorance is not an absence of knowledge, but an active turning from Truth. It is a spiritual blindness in which you close your own eyes and literally ignore what is before you. Spiritual awakening occurs when you open your eyes to what is, and what always has been, right in front of you. This awakening is yours to accomplish. You must put forth the effort.

It is not a question of effort as opposed to surrender. Ignorance, Egoism, Desire, Aversion, and Clinging must be surrendered. Let them go! If conceiving of giving them to some higher power helps then by all means do so. Do not, however, think that you can escape working on yourself and applying effort. Changing habits of Misery into those of Joy takes effort. Joy may leap forth of its own accord, but impediments must first be moved aside.

As you practice you will learn that letting go and effort go hand in hand. They are opposites only conceptually. When your mind is still and all words have melted into silence, you will recognize your Truth!

APPENDIX A

A Meditation Exercise

The heart of meditation is concentration on a single thought, image, sound, etc. A focus of concentration may be very narrow, e.g., a blue light inside your head, or it may be quite broad, e.g., keeping your mind on the road and its traffic while driving. In meditation it is customary to keep your focus narrow.

There are many ways to meditate depending on the object chosen and the posture assumed. Here I present a relatively simple approach, a method good for beginners and experienced meditators alike. You can practice it for the rest of your life.

Don't concern yourself with whether or not you are a beginner or an "advanced" student of meditation. Such concepts have no relevance when it comes to actual practice. My teacher once stated that all students, beginners and more experienced, are simply working to pull the weeds from their mental gardens. All will need to keep at it until their karma is exhausted.

You need a place to practice. The most important aspect is to minimize interruptions from other people. This can be difficult if you live in a family and your quarters are small. You may need to adjust your schedule so that you can find a time when others are still sleeping or not at home.

Although it is desirable, you do not need a separate room for meditation. You can use a corner of a bedroom or study. For a number of years I used the living room as a place to practice postures and made sure to arise at least an hour before anyone else. When others got up I went into the bedroom to sit in meditation.

Some suggest that you construct a kind of altar where you meditate. It can contain a statue, a picture of a teacher, or simply some flowers. The idea is that the place where you meditate and the objects on the altar serve as cues that evoke the appropriate mood when you begin. The other side of the coin is that you might become attached to the place and the objects and not be able to meditate without them. In my opinion it is best to keep things simple and not risk the added attachments.

Ideally, family members will respect what you are trying to do. If you have small children, however, this may not be the case. Children are egocentric by nature and may not be able to appreciate your need for quiet. Also, as a parent you have a responsibility to meet their needs. You may have to make compromises. Yelling at your kids when they interrupt your meditation harms both them and you.

Finding a noise free environment may be hard if you live in a city. As you progress in your practice, however, you will learn to find *internal silence* even when external noise is present. If your place is noisy learn to listen for the silent spaces within or between the noises. All sound arises from a silence that is ever-present within. Learn to fall into that silence. Meditation is essentially an *inward* process, the cultivation of internal quiet regardless of what is going on around you. This is a tall order, but others have done it so you can as well.

You need to adopt a comfortable "seat" for meditation. A firm mat can do for both meditation and posture work. You may also need a cushion under your buttocks and/or knees if you are going to sit cross-legged and are not used to a sitting posture. For a long time I folded an old mattress pad on the bedroom floor. Eventually I added a *zafu*, a cushion favored by Zen Buddhists. After many years the mattress pad disintegrated and I sprang for a so-called "sticky mat" from a commercial yoga supply house. These rubber mats come in a variety of widths and are easy to fold in half when necessary. They also roll easily for transport. If you have a teacher s/he should be a source of helpful advice about equipment. As with altars, however, I would try to keep equipment to a minimum.

One item you may find useful is a timer so that you will not be concerned about time while meditating. I used to use a solid-state watch with a countdown timer. Now I use an inexpensive solid-state timer that I purchased at a Radio Shack. The time out sound is not too raucous. It is possible to buy sophisticated meditation timers that make a pleasant gong like sound. These tend to be very expensive, however.

Whatever kind of timer you choose set it initially for ten or 15 minutes. After three or five sessions add five more minutes. Gradually, at a pace that suits you, increase the time to 30 minutes. I would not exceed 40 minutes without a break. If you wish to meditate for a longer period I suggest you alternate 25 minutes of meditating with ten or 15 minutes of exercise, either walking or postures involving leg stretches, etc. As I have said before, it is best to have a teacher to guide you in these matters. One size does not always fit all.

What posture should you adopt for meditation? Know first that a firm "seat" does not necessarily imply a seated posture. It refers to the disposition of your mind. Posture is important, however, for the attitude of the body directly reflects and influences your mental attitude. First, you need to be relaxed and comfortable, but not slouching. Ideally your back, neck and head should be in proper alignment so that your spine is straight, but not rigid. This can be achieved either in a traditional cross-legged pose, sitting in a straight-backed chair, or lying on your back on a mat on the floor as in the dead pose (corpse posture). You can also meditate standing up as is sometimes done in *taijiquan.*

When asked what was the most important yoga posture Ramana Maharshi once responded, "Concentration!" Whether sitting, standing, or lying on your back, it is the quality of concentration that makes your "seat" firm and proper.

Unless you are already accomplished at some sitting pose such as *padmasana* (lotus posture) or *siddhasana* (adept's posture) I suggest you start by lying on your back with your feet stretched out in front of you and your arms at your side with your palms facing up. This is the dead pose or corpse posture (*savasana*). Lie on a firm mat or folded blanket so that you don't lose body heat into the floor. Do not lie on a bed, sofa, or other surface that is overly soft. Sleep habits will be much more intense under those circumstances.

Once you are comfortable in the posture, become aware of the natural rhythm of your breathing, evenly in and evenly out. Every time you breathe out feel yourself give way and "sink" into the mat. As you breathe evenly in and out select some spot on the ceiling above you (more or less above your chest or belly) and let your eyes come to rest on that spot. Try not to stare at it, but literally *rest* your eyes.

You do not have to breathe in any special way other than to observe the natural rhythm of breathing in and out. You may become aware of the movement of your abdomen, the feeling of breath through your nostrils, or some other natural aspect of your breathing. Whatever it may be let your mind make a *pleasing* connection with that sensory object.

With your eyes still open and resting on the spot above you, count down slowly (there is no hurry) from ten to zero. When you reach zero close your eyes and simply allow your mind to rest on the natural rhythm of your breathing in and out.

If you should feel the need to sigh, cough, or clear your throat feel free to do so. Just observe what is taking place without making any judgments. No one is going to grade you on this.

Keep trying to rest your attention on your breathing. As you breathe in try to get a feeling of becoming increasingly awake and aware. Do not worry, however, if you feel sleepy at first. If you should fall asleep while doing this exercise there is no shame in it, only know that sleep is not meditation. With practice you will find that if you do doze off you soon awaken feeling refreshed and alert.

As you breathe out shift to a feeling of letting go. Each time you exhale feel yourself give way and "melt" into the mat beneath you.

After a few minutes of observing your breathing you may find yourself distracted by thoughts arising in your mind or by sounds in your room or outside. Your mind may begin to drift toward issues and problems of your life and feel a need to keep working on them. Do not attempt to interfere in any direct way with this tendency. In other words do not trouble with trouble or get into a battle with your own mind. Instead, as soon as you notice that you have drifted, bring your attention back to your breathing. As long as you keep coming back to your breathing you will be fine.

Waste no effort whatsoever in judging yourself when you become distracted. Self-criticism does nothing but complicate the situation and expand the distraction. You need only do one thing and that is keep bringing your mind back to rest on the natural rhythm of your breathing.

Do not get caught up in wondering how well you are doing. Such judgment games are a distraction. They represent the work of the ego getting itself into competition and/or comparison. For example, you may find that you entertain fancies of being a saint, monk, or great yogi. Great yogis aren't concerned with being "great". They no longer even concern themselves with enlightenment and ignorance. They simply are fully awake and practice for the sake of practice.

Therefore, rest your mind on the rhythm of your breathing in and breathing out. Learn to be fully here. Every time you breathe out get the feeling of letting go. Always keep letting go and know that you can always let go a little bit more.

As for any problems and questions you really do need to find yourself a teacher. Practice, persevere, and good luck!

APPENDIX B

Suggested Reading

The works listed below are some I have found helpful in the course of my studies. None of them is a substitute for actual practice under the mentorship of a teacher. Reading them, however, is a form of concentration. It orients and directs your mind toward freedom within.

Some may no longer be in print. I trust, however, that you can find them in libraries or used bookstores.

The list is not alphabetized, but arranged in an order that appeals to my way of thinking about the subject matter.

Feuerstein, Georg. *The Yoga Tradition*. Hohm Press: Prescott, Arizona, 1998. An excellent history of yoga practice and theory. It also contains a useful glossary.

_____. *The Yoga-Sutra of Patanjali*. Inner Traditions: Rochester, Vermont, 1989. Georg Feuerstein is a Sanskrit scholar, student of philosophy and anthropology, and long time practitioner of several forms of yoga. Although I sometimes find his writing more transcendentalist than I care for, he is a serious student of the subject and has an encyclopedic grasp of its literature. This translation of the *Yogasutra* is one of the best.

Aranya, Swami Hariharananda. *Yoga Philosophy of Patanjali*. State University of New York Press: Albany, New York, 1983. It is always good to read more than one translation of a work. In my own researches I have used about six translations of the *Yogasutra* and found them to differ in significant ways. Don't let this disturb you. The more the "experts" disagree the more there is room for your own interpretation. This volume contains what I understand is a good translation of Vyasa's commentary on the aphorisms. As far as I know this was the original commentary composed around 500 B.C.E. Modern commentaries are worth studying, but too often reflect Western cultural biases.

Coster, Geraldine. *Yoga and Western Psychology: A Comparison*. Oxford U. Press: London, 1934. This is the first modern psychological work on the

Yogasutra I ever read and it has a sentimental value for me. It contains yet another rendering of the *Yogasutra* as well as an interpretation from the point of view of psychodynamic psychology *a la* the 1930's.

Nikhilananda, Swami. *The Principal Upanishads.* Dover: Mineola, N.Y., 2003. The Upanishads are pretty basic and contain much that is fundamental to the development of yoga psychology. The ideas introduced belong primarily to the traditions of *jnana* yoga (the yoga of self-knowledge) and *dhyana* yoga (the yoga of meditation). Although I include only this one translation it would be wise to take a look at others as well.

Purohit, Swami. *The Geeta.* Faber and Faber: London, 1935. If there is a Hindu "bible" this is it. The *Bhagavad Gita* is the most revered scripture of the Hindu collection. It introduces *karma* yoga (action without attachment to the consequences) and *bhakti* yoga (devotion or surrender to a deity). The two may be combined when one surrenders the fruits of action to a deity. This translation is by a man who, I understand, was at one time guru to the poet William Butler Yeats.

Sinha, Pulgenda. *The Gita As It Was.* Open Court: La Salle, Illinois, 1986. Sinha makes the claim that current translations of the *Bhagavad Gita* contain theistic interpolations that do not represent the *Samkhya* rationalist approach of the original. I find his argument convincing. The result is a translation of the "original" Gita without the usual monistic theological emphasis.

Maharshi, Ramana. *Talks With Ramana Maharshi.* Inner Directions: Carlsbad, California, 2000. Ken Wilber called Maharshi "…the greatest living sage of the twentieth century." I often don't agree with Wilber (much too transcendental and intellectual for my taste), but I do on this. If I had to give away all of my books but one this is the one I would keep. Buy it, read it over and over. Then go practice accordingly.

Godman, David. *The Teachings of Sri Ramana Maharshi.* Godman has edited Maharshi's oral teachings and arranged them in order of their listener's readiness to hear them. This may be the best introduction to Maharshi in print.

Waddell, Norman, and Abe, Masao. *The Heart of Dogen's Shobogenzo.* State University of New York Press: Albany, New York, 2002. Dogen, the founder of the Soto school of Zen Buddhism, has been called a religious genius. While Ramana Maharshi wore nothing more than a loin cloth and lived near the foot of a sacred mountain in Southern India during the twentieth century, Dogen was a fully robed priest and master within the confines of institutional Buddhism in thirteenth century Japan. Both, however, learned to ride the same ox even if they then returned to somewhat different villages. Either one can show you how to go naked into the world. Reading Maharshi will help you understand Dogen.

Guenon, Rene. *Man and His Becoming According to the Vedanta*. Noonday Press: New York, 1958. For those who can't do without metaphysics this is one of the best presentations of *Vedanta* philosophy I know.

Bernard, Theos. *Heaven Lies Within Us*. Scribner's: New York, 1939. A personal account of Bernard's encounter with yogic practice and philosophy. It is relatively free of the sentimentalism that usually infects such accounts. Bernard was a true practitioner and not an academic dilettante although he did acquire academic credentials in the area. It is my understanding that Bernard was the first American to receive initiation in Tibet from actual lamas. This occurred in 1936-37 and is recounted in his book, *Penthouse of the Gods*.

Krishnamurti, J. *This Light in Oneself: True Meditation*. Shambhala: Boston, 1999. This will give you a somewhat different slant on the nature of meditation. It is a good antedote to getting "uptight" about it.

Bharati, Agehananda. *The Light at the Center: Context and Pretext in Modern Mysticism*. Ross-Erikson: Santa Barbara, CA, 1976. This provides a useful, if at times acerbic, counter to the overly romantic interpretations of Eastern spiritual practices that arose during the 1970's and '80's and still abound in much transpersonal and New Age literature.

APPENDIX C

Glossary

This presents key terms used in the text. When a term is the equivalent (or an approximation) to a *Sanskrit* (Skt.) word that word is given either in parentheses or used as part of the definition/discussion. These definitions are not necessarily those agreed to by scholars, but represent how I use the terms. If a word in a definition is also listed in the glossary it is in **bold face**. For another glossary see Feurstein, Georg in Appendix B. Suggested Reading.

Absolute (or The Absolute): That which is Real, i.e., permanent and independent of any conditions. The Absolute is not dependent on relationships with any objects or processes. The Absolute is not subject to birth and death. It is "deathless" and "unborn". Words cannot describe the Absolute. It is best represented by silence. Conceptually the Absolute stands in opposition to the **relative** and the ever-changing world of **nature and experience**. In yoga and **Vedanta** philosophy the Absolute is called *Brahman*.

Absorption (*Samadhi*): A stage of concentration in which mental process is completely involved with its chosen object and nothing else intrudes. Absorption may be either with or without seed, i.e., an object. Regarding the latter see also **emptiness** and **open space**.

Actual, actuality: Refers to experience directly evoked by sensory activity as opposed to **fancy**, experience evoked by words alone. Actual knowledge or actual reality is distinguished from **virtual** knowledge or reality.

Atman: A Sanskrit term for one's **True Self-nature**. The *Atman* is *Brahman* residing as the True Self-nature of a person. *Atman* is identical with *Brahman*, and cannot be described in words. Qualities cannot be attributed to either *Atman* or *Brahman*.

Aversion: One of the five **sources of affliction**; a cause of Misery. Aversion is defined as a preoccupation with pain, avoidance, and defensiveness. You might think of it as the "flip side" of **Desire**.

Avidya: The Sanskrit word for **ignorance** of one's **True Self-nature**, and therefore the primary source of affliction and Misery. The Indo-European root *vid* is etymologically related to the "vis" in vision, the "wis" in wisdom, and the "wiz" in wizard. Thus *avidya* is a form of "spiritual blindness", i.e., not seeing the truth of one's own nature.

Bodhisattva: A Buddhist term for a person who has developed spiritually to the point where s/he could "enter" Nirvana, but out of compassion for others remains in "this world" to assist them in finding release from suffering.

Brahman: A Sanskrit word designating the **absolute,** or ultimate reality. *Brahman* is without conditions and cannot be described in words. According to **Vedanta** teaching, *Brahman* may only be described as pure **Being**, Consciousness, and Bliss, and has no other properties or attributes. As used here *Brahman* is conceived as pure Being such that all existence is *Brahman* and nothing exists apart from *Brahman*. *Brahman* should not be equated with a personal deity, creator, or savior. If one has to theologize *Brahman* Meister Eckhart's Godhead comes close.

Brahminism: The religion of the *Brahmin* or priestly caste of orthodox Hinduism. Brahminism has its roots in the **Vedas** and is associated with secret priestly knowledge and ritual sacrifice.

Breath control: (*pranayama*) An umbrella term referring to any of a number of techniques for regulating the breath. It refers to the fourth of the eight limbs of the "**tree of yoga**" as described by **Patanjali**. The Sanskrit word *pranayama* implies control of *prana* or "vital energy".

Carelessness: One of the **obstacles** that impede spiritual progress and practice. Carelessness is an impairment of both thought and action. It can range from illogical and uncritical thinking, through lack of attention to detail, to sloppy and awkward execution of actions.

Chakra:A Sanskrit term that literally means "wheel" and is commonly used to denote "energy centers" in the body. According to Agehananda Bharati (see suggested reading) the *chakras* are **imaginal** and their description in the **tantric** literature is intended to provide objects for meditation. Some recent writers have attempted to link the *chakras* to the ways in which human beings experience their bodily processes, emotions, etc.

Classical yoga: Following Feuerstein (see Appendix B. Sugested Reading) this term refers to the system presented in the *Yogasutra of Patanjali*. The emphasis in this system is on psychological training, i.e., the use of concentration to quiet mental process. See also the **eight limbs of yoga**.

Clinging (to mundane existence): One of the five **sources of affliction**. Clinging is the fifth source of affliction also known as the **fear of death**. It is the psychological extension of **ignorance** and **egoism** and represents the full flowering of **aversion**.

Concentration (*ekagrata*): Keeping the mind on one point, i.e., one-pointed concentration. As a meditative discipline it refers to the establishment of a pleasing connection of the mind with an object. The word "pleasing" stands in contrast to the concept of concentration as something forced, artificial, and therefore unpleasant. With practice concentration becomes effortless and the practitioner is drawn to it. It is important to understand that the focus of concentration can be narrow (a single syllable *mantram*) or broad (reading yogic literature).

Conceptualization: The principal subclass of **fancy**. Conceptualization is a class of knowledge evoked by words rather than direct sensory activity. Conceptualizations are abstractions, i.e., concept labels that do not denote **actual** objects. When their true nature is not perceived they can produce verbal delusion, a cognitive state in which a conceptualization is treated as an actual object.

Crystal Clarity: A cognitive condition or state of consciousness dominated by **Truth**, one of the three **qualities** of **nature and experience**. When mental process is dominated by Clarity or **Truth** you can "see things as they are", i.e., you can see "what is".

Desire: One of the five **sources of affliction**. Desire is rooted in **egoism** and defined as a preoccupation or entanglement with pleasure. Desire sets the stage for **aversion** and is a major cause of **misery**.

Desirelessness (*vairagya*): Desirelessness is a *feeling of inward mastery* that comes from letting go of the thirst for both material and spiritual attainments. The Sanskrit term is usually translated as "dispassion", but to my mind that word is too suggestive of a lack of feeling and emotion that fails to convey the psychological import of the term.

Discrimination: The cognitive capacity or process of distinguishing one thing from another including self from other. It involves the making or constructing of differences. The discriminative capacity makes the perception of distinct objects possible including the distinguishing of figure from ground. Without the capacity for discrimination the delusion of **separation** could not take root. The ability to discriminate is not dependent upon language as some contend (e.g., the immune system discriminates self from other), but is greatly enhanced through language via naming and classifying.

Discriminative wisdom (*prajna, jnana*): The "process" or "power" of seeing Truth or "seeing through" veils of delusion. It is the wisdom that discriminates Truth from delusion and falsehood.

Disease: More appropriately, dis-ease or a lack of satisfaction with life in general. While the term includes physical illness, the emphasis is upon psychical or psychological dis-ease. It involves a sense that things are not as they should be. This usually means that things are not as you would prefer them to be.

Distracted: A state in which you cannot maintain concentration on an intended single point because attention is drawn to another point, e.g., some fantasy. Compare to **fickle-minded**.

Dualistic thinking: Dualistic thinking construes experience in terms of opposites, up v. down, right v. wrong, self v. other, and perpetuates the delusion of **separation**. Dualistic thinking supports adversarial and competitive processes.

Ego function (*ahamkara*): The ego function is the cognitive capacity to separate self from other, i.e., the capacity for self-consciousness. It is a prerequisite for, but should not to be confused with, **egoism**.

Egoism: The perception (and feeling) of ownership of, and identification with, the body. Egoism is one of the five **sources of affliction**. See also **great knot**.

Eight limbs of yoga (*ashtanga yoga*): The process of yoga is likened to a tree with eight limbs, i.e., practices. These are: **restraints**, **observances**, **posture**, **breath control**, **withdrawal of the senses**, **fixed attention**, **meditation**, and **absorption**.

Emptiness: As used in this work emptiness refers to **absorption** without an object, i.e., mental process is "empty". This is different from the Buddhist concept of emptiness or *sunyata*, i.e., that all things lack inherent essence or "self". *Sunyata* is, however, related to the yogic assertion that all things in nature and experience are ephemeral, i.e., impermanent. See also **open space**.

Energy (*rajas*): One of the three basic **qualities** or "moods" of **nature and experience**. Energy refers to experiences of dynamism, activity, vigorous movement, etc. Its psychopathological extreme is mania.

Faith: As used here faith refers not to any set of beliefs or a creed, but to an inward sense of trust arising from the cultivation of **desirelessness**. It implies a willingness to "leap into the void" or let go.

Fancy. A class of knowledge or experience not supported by sensory activity, but arising from words alone. The most common form of fancy is **conceptualization.** Other forms are dreams and hallucinations. A classic example of fancy is "the 'horns' of the hare".

Fear of death: See **clinging**.

Fickle-minded: A state of mind in which concentration is not maintained because the mind darts from one object to another. Fickle-minded mental thinking is tangential in nature. Compare to **distracted**.

Fixed attention (*dharana*): A stage of the **inner discipline** in which the practitioner, while keeping mental process focused on a single object or thought, is conscious of the effort to do so.

Granthi: Sanskrit word meaning "knot". Refers to stoppages or blockages of the natural flow of energy in the body. See **great knot** below.

Great knot: A metaphoric image of one's identification with the body. This identification is a primary aspect of **egoism** and is prerequisite for **desire, aversion**, and the **fear of death**. The fears and anxieties generated by these **sources of affliction** "tie one in knots" and prevent a free, creative, and spontaneous enjoyment of life.

Gross objects: Mental objects (thoughts, ideas, perceptions, cognitions) that are readily accessible parts of one's personal narrative, world view, or internal conversations. Gross objects represent the relatively "surface" or "shallow" levels of the body of individual consciousness. Closest Sanskrit term may be *vitarka*. See also **subtle objects**.

Hatha **yoga**: Developed in connection with **tantra**, *hatha* yoga views the human body as a microcosm of the universal macrocosm so that when properly trained it becomes a vehicle of release from **misery**. *Hatha* may be translated as "force" or "forceful" because its practices are relatively strenuous and aimed at forcing the *kundalini* energy into and up the central channel (*susumna nadi*) to the crown chakra (*sahasrara*). The syllable "*ha*" refers to sun or male energy and "*tha*" to moon or female energy such that the word *hatha* represents the union of these energies. In today's popular culture the term *hatha yoga* is normally used to refer only to systems of postures and breathing exercises practiced for health and fitness. In the present work the term refers to the system of bodily discipline that is accessory to and supportive of the practice of **concentration**.

Ignorance (*avidya*): Ignorance is the first of the five **sources of affliction** and the foundation for the others: **egoism, desire, aversion**, and **clinging to mundane reality** (fear of death). Ignorance is not an absence of knowledge, but an active process of ignoring or turning a blind eye to one's **True Self-nature**. Another term for Ignorance is **spiritual blindness**.

Imaginal. This adjective is used instead of "imaginary" to avoid implications of triviality, e.g., that a thing is "only" imaginary. The experience of the imaginal is anything but trivial and often reflects the entry into personal consciousness of transpersonal or collective content. Imaginal experiences can be of great significance to the psychic life of an individual. They are, however, still experiences and thus essentially ephemeral. Preoccupation with them can be a powerful distraction from practice.

Imagination: The power to produce or conjure images. This power is fundamental to the construction of all experience, actual and virtual.

Indecision: The inability to make up your mind. Indecision is expressed in hesitancy and awkwardness. Indecision is one of the **obstacles** that arise from the **sources of affliction**.

Inertia (*tamas*): One of the three **qualities** or moods of **nature and experience**. Inertia denotes experiences of mass, weight, solidity, opacity, sluggishness, depression, etc.

Inner discipline: the inner discipline includes the limbs of the **tree of yoga** that follow **withdrawal of the senses**, i.e., **fixed attention**, **meditation**, and **absorption**. See also **outer discipline**.

Instability: Not being able to maintain concentration. You can get started, but can't stick with it. Instability is one of the **obstacles**.

Karma: The universal law of cause and effect that states that all events are caused, and all actions have consequences (effects). Classical theory argues that every action leaves a karmic residue, i.e., traces, within the mind. This residue functions as a "storehouse" of "seeds" that may or may not bear fruit depending on conditions. Modern versions of the karmic doctrine include behaviorism's Law of Effect, family therapy's cross-generational transmission, genetics, and explanations of "traces" in terms of neural circuitry, e.g., synaptic modification.

Knots (*granthi*): Knots represent blockages of the natural flow of psychophysical energy in the body-mind complex. They may be related to repressed feelings, miseducation, fears, inhibitions, etc. They also represent anxiety driven points of clinging and fears of letting go. See **great knot**.

Koan: A Japanese version of the Chinese word *kung-an* that means, roughly, "case". Koans are questions or puzzles used as foci for meditation in Zen Buddhism. Their aim is to "tie-up" the thinking mind with an unsolvable problem, thus sowing "great doubt" and ultimately leading to letting go of dependency on reason to resolve spiritual issues.

Kriya yoga: Yoga of action. The principal actions are **practice** and the cultivation of **desirelessness**.

Kundalini shakti: Sometimes referred to as the "serpent power", *kundalini* is conceived as a force or energy lying dormant (like a coiled serpent) near the *muladhara chakra* at the base of the *susumna* (central channel).

Kundalini yoga: The use of **hatha yoga** and other practices to arouse the ***kundalini shakti***.

Kungfuzi: Pinyin spelling of Confucius.

Languor: A lack of energy, enthusiasm, or motivation. Languor is one of the **obstacles**.

Laziness: A felt sense of inner "heaviness". There are things you want to do, but a feeling of inward "heaviness" weighs you down. Laziness is one of the **obstacles**.

Lingam-yoni yoga: The use of sexual intercourse in yoga. *Lingam* refers to the male organ and *yoni* to the female.

Mantram: A syllable, word, phrase, or longer passage repeated over and over as a focus for meditative concentration. In Sanskrit *mantra* is plural and *mantram* singular.

Meditation (*dhyana*): A state of consciousness in which mental process is focused on a single thought or object, but unlike **fixed attention** (*dharana*) the feeling of effort has been let go. There does remain a sense of self-conscious intent, i.e., "I am doing this". Such concentration is thus not yet free of ego.

Memory: A cognitive process in which representations or images of past events are "held onto". In yoga psychology it is the action of *holding* to the past that is emphasized as opposed to concern with mechanisms of recall, recollection, or reconstruction.

Mindfulness: In Buddhism mindfulness refers to the process of maintaining "bare" attention to the present moment. This includes detached observation of one's own inward and outward activities. Mindfulness has been contrasted with concentrative meditation in that mindfulness theoretically employs no special focus while concentration does involve a focus. In my view this distinction is too simplistic and ignores the complexities of actual practice and experience.

Misconception: Entertaining a false view of something. Clinging to wrong knowledge. Misconception is one of the **obstacles**.

Misery: Suffering in all its forms. Misery refers to the entire range of human experiences of discomfort, unpleasantness, vexation, frustration, embarrassment, pain, fear, anxiety, *ad nauseum*.

Missing the point: A failure to concentrate or stay on point. Includes not being able to follow an argument or line of evidence to a valid conclusion. If you miss the point you just don't "get it". Missing the point is one of the **obstacles**.

Muladhara chakra: The "root" *chakra* or energy center located at the base of the central channel or ***susumna***. It has been identified with the perineal area between the anus and the genitalia.

Nature and experience: The realm of experience. This includes the totality of all that is experienced or can be experienced. All experiences have beginnings and endings, i.e., are ephemeral and subject to birth and death. This means that all objects of sensory, perceptual, and cognitive process are entirely relative and impermanent. Nature and experience is sometimes also called the realm of name and form or the realm of the senses.

Nirvana: The word literally means something like "blowing out" as in extinguishing the flame of a candle. Modern yoga psychology therefore views nirvana as the *cessation* of the processes that cause Misery. In contemporary **transpersonal psychology** the tendency has been to view *nirvana* as a positive state or condition.

Observances (*niyama*): The observances constitute the second limb of the **tree of yoga**. They are: cleanliness (internal and external), contentment, austerity, study, and devotion to the "lord" (an image of one who has worked successfully to get free of **misery**).

Obstacles: The obstacles are the basic miseries that emanate from the five **sources of affliction** and stand in the way of living a life of free and spontaneous enjoyment. They are **disease, languor, laziness, indecision, carelessness, sensuality, misconception, missing the point**, and **instability**.

Open space: When there is **absorption** without an object the mind no longer clings to anything but is "open" or presents an "open space". This term is employed in translating some Tibetan Buddhist texts, but I am not sure my usage is the same.

Outer discipline: The outer discipline encompasses the first four limbs of the **tree of yoga**, i.e., **restraints, observances, posture**, and **breath control**. See also **inner discipline** and **withdrawal of the senses**.

Patanjali: The name given to the author-compiler of the *Yogasutra*. His actual identity is not known, but tradition identifies him with a famous second century grammarian of that name.

Posture (*asana*): The third limb of the **tree of yoga** and part of the **outer discipline**. The practice of physical postures is intended to support breathing exercises as well as the practices of the **inner discipline**. The point is to develop a firm and stable sitting posture, bodily strength and endurance, and flexibility. The outer bodily discipline functions to establish mental attitudes conducive to practicing the inner discipline.

Practice: Any effort to steady the mind.

Prakriti: Literally, "creatrix" (i.e., Mother Nature). In **samkhya's** dualistic philosophy *prakriti* represents the realm of pure matter, i.e., the realm of **nature**

and experience. As such it is the "seen" that exists solely for the enjoyment of the "seer", i.e., *purusha*.

Purusha: Traditional yoga and *Samkhya* term for "Self" or spirit. In **samkhya** philosophy it represents the male or spiritual aspect of the cosmic duality as opposed to the material (see **prakriti**). Note that "spirit" should not be taken to refer to a ghost or other entity belonging to a supposed spirit realm.

Qualities (of **nature and experience**): The qualities refer to the three *gunas*: *sattva* (**truth**), *rajas* (**energy**), and *tamas* (**inertia**). These *gunas* are traditionally conceived as the basic constituents of material nature. Here they are presented as "moods" reflected in all experience. See individual entries for each quality.

Raja yoga: Literally, "king of yogas" or "kingly yoga". The term is usually used to refer to the system of yoga described in the *Yogasutra of Patanjali*.

Relative: That which is relative depends upon relationships with other entities, i.e., various causes and conditions. It is also referred to as "conditional". Relative things have no absolute self-nature or essence. Relative things are subject to change; they are not permanent. All things relative are subject to coming and going, birth and death.

Restraints (*yama*): The first of the eight limbs of yoga. The restraints represent self-discipline and are five in number: nonviolence (doing no harm), truthfulness (not lying to one's self and others), not stealing, letting go of lust, letting go of greed.

Sadhu(s): Individuals who have dedicated their lives to spiritual practice (*sadhana*).

Sahasrara: The uppermost of the *chakras* or centers of psychic energy. Usually described as located at the crown of the head, hence its other name, "crown chakra". Some sources locate it just above the crown, which could suggest independence from the body, i.e., severing of the **great knot**.

Samadhi: see **Absorption**.

Samkhya: A philosophy postulating a dualism of pure spirit as "seer" (*purusha*) and a realm of pure matter (*prakriti*), i.e., the realm of nature and experience as that which is "seen". *Samkhya* has been claimed to be the world's oldest philosophy.

Sangha(s): A group of practitioners, yogis, or monks, meeting together.

Seeing through: I use this term to denote the activity of **discriminative wisdom** (*prajna*) in discerning Truth from falsehood and delusion. It refers to seeing through the "smoke" of **Ignorance**. In colloquial terms, being able to "see through" means having a good "crap" detector.

Seen, the: The realm of **nature and experience** (*Prakriti*). See also the **seer**.

Seer, the: Another term for **Purusha**, as **True Self** or absolute subject.

Sensuality: Attachment to objects of sensory pleasure, e.g., lust and gluttony.

Separation: A delusion in which self is perceived as separate from other. This delusion casts a dark shadow on all human cognition as long as it is allowed to function.

Sexual energy: In yoga psychology this refers to **Shakti** or generative energy. It is not limited to sexual intercourse, but extends to all manner of creative activity.

Shadow: This has two meanings depending on context. In modern yoga psychology the delusion of **separation** is held to cast a "shadow" over human consciousness that leads to **ignorance**. "Shadow" is also a term in the psychology of C. G. Jung and refers to psychic content, e.g., experiences, feelings, and imagery disowned by the personal egocentric consciousness. The two usages are related in that the delusion of separation produces anxiety that leads to its repression. In Jungian terms it might be said that the feeling/perception of separation is relegated to the domain of the shadow. Although repressed the delusion of separation still manages to cast its own shadow upon our mental lives.

Shakti: In **Shaivism** and **Tantra,** Shakti names the generative feminine energy responsible for creation. This energy also operates in the human body and its harnessing is one of the aims of **hatha yoga**. When referring to the arousing of this otherwise dormant or blocked energy by means of yoga it is referred to as **kundalini shakti**.

Shaivism: In Hinduism, a complex of beliefs and practices centering on **Shiva** as the primary manifestation or image of the Absolute.

Shaman: A person supposedly possessing the ability to travel to or communicate with alternate realities (e.g., the "spirit realm") in the interests of influencing events in this world. In most cultures shamanism is associated with healing and prognostication, but its practices run the gamut of both "white" and "black" magic. According to some accounts shamans can shape-shift, i.e., assume animal forms in order to carry out their tasks. Modern accounts tend to emphasize shamanic practices (drumming, chanting, ingesting psychedelic substances) as techniques for altering consciousness.

Shiva: In the Hindu pantheon *Shiva* is the god of destruction. *Shiva* is not negative or malevolent, but manifests the need to destroy (let go of) one form in order to bring another into existence. As the god of yoga, *Shiva* is a destroyer of **ignorance** and its spawn. In **Shaivism** *Shiva* is supreme lord of the universe, but not its creator. Creation is carried out through the generative action of **Shakti**, the female energy or goddess, once the seed has been sown in a cosmic coupling with Shiva. These cosmic energies or forces should not be identified with human genders. All human beings, male and female, potentially embody both *Shiva* and *Shakti* in so far as they can let go and lead naturally generative lives.

Siddhis: Supposedly paranormal powers acquired as the result of practicing yoga. In this text I have suggested that the *siddhis* may be conceived as **imaginal** powers. As such they represent feats of the creative imagination made possible when previously habitual modes of perceiving are let go.

Soto Zen: A sect of Zen Buddhism that advocates sitting meditation (*zazen*) with an attitude of "sitting just to sit". The idea, as I understand it, is that one does not practice *in order* to attain anything, but to be fully present to "what already is". As I see it, this is akin to yoga's carrying out **practice** in a spirit of **desirelessness**.

Sources of Affliction (*klesas*): The five sources are **ignorance, egoism, desire, aversion**, and **clinging to mundane existence** (also called the **fear of death**). They constitute the causes of **misery**.

Spiritual blindness (*avidya*): See **Ignorance**.

Subtle body (*linga sharira*): Contrasted with the gross, physical, or material body, the subtle body includes the animating properties that bring the gross body to life. In modern yoga psychology subtle body refers to the *experience* of energy functions, feelings and emotions, imagery and representational process, as well as higher intellectual processes and awareness. Attachment to the subtle body is as much an aspect of **egoism** as attachment to the gross body. Attachment itself is a subtle process.

Subtle objects: Mental objects (thoughts, ideas, perceptions, cognitions) that are usually unconscious and take special work to reveal. These need not be repressed contents, but can include assumptions, beliefs, and rules that guide or structure mental process. Jungian archetypes might be one example. At a "deeper" (less readily accessible) level of subtlety are the categories of space, time, and cause. The best *Sanskrit* equivalent might be **vichara**. See also **gross objects**.

Susumna: The central channel (*nadi*) in the Tantric "anatomical" system.

Tantra: Literally means "ancient text". Also carries the connotation of continuity or a "thread" that runs through the "fabric" of existence. Tantra is a collection of teachings that emphasizes the non-duality of sacred and profane domains. In its theistic forms worship of feminine or earth energy is emphasized. Tantra views the human body as a microcosmic reflection or emanation of the macrocosm and a vehicle for achieving release from Misery. This latter view has been important in the development of **hatha** yoga.

Tantric yoga: Any yogic practice directly informed by tantric principles. Tantric yoga emphasizes use of the body as a vehicle for achieving release from **misery**. Traditional *hatha* **yoga** is a form of tantric yoga as is *kundalini* **yoga**. The use of **mantra**, **yantra**, and visualization is common. Tantric yoga is not restricted to sexual practices and may be carried out without engaging in sexual intercourse.

Transpersonal psychology: A modern outgrowth of humanistic psychology with special interest in altered states of consciousness, religious and peak experiences, and the investigation of spiritual practices. Some transpersonal psychologists are also interested in parapsychology.

Tree of yoga: Refers to the corpus of *Patanajali's yoga* conceived as a tree with eight limbs (ashta-anga). Each limb represents a domain of practice: **observances** (*yama*), **restraints** (*niyama*), **posture** (*asana*), **breath control** (*pranayama*), **withdrawal of the senses** (*pratyahara*), **fixed attention** (*dharana*), **meditation** (*dhyana*), and **absorption** (*samadhi*). See also, **outer discipline** and **inner discipline**.

True Self-nature: See *Atman*.

Truth: One of the three **qualities** or moods of **nature and experience**. Also called "clarity". When the mind is dominated by clarity it can apprehend the Truth, i.e., see things as they truly are. Truth is the quality most natural to mental process. Ideally, a clear mind reflects and reveals "what is". Unfortunately, mind can also be dominated by **Energy** or **Inertia** in which case mental clarity is disturbed or obscured. It is also important to realize that one can make a condition of "clarity" an object of **desire** and attachment.

Uncomplicated calm: A state in which mental process is free of complications caused by clinging or attachment. The mental space may be either empty or steady and flowing. In the latter case mental process flows calmly without self-reflective "knotting". The result is a conflict free state. See also **emptiness**.

Upanishads: A body of Hindu literature that is highly important for the study of yoga. The word itself conveys the image of a student sitting at the feet of a teacher thus emphasizing the importance of direct and personal mentoring. The first *Upanishads* may have been transmitted around 1500 B.C.E. The major *Upanishads* emphasize the identity of *Brahman* and *Atman*, thus teaching that a person's **True Self-nature** is identical with the **Absolute**. The *Upanishads* introduced the yogas of *jnana* (self knowledge) and *dhyana* (meditation). Since many of the teachers depicted in the *Upanishads* were of the ruling or warrior caste they represent a departure from reliance on priestly authority and ritual in favor of self-discipline and personal inward inquiry.

Vedanta: Literally "end of the *Vedas.*" Vedanta is a body of teaching that claims roots in the *Vedas* and, according to some, represents the pinnacle of that tradition. Non-dual *Vedanta* argued that ultimate reality was "not two" as opposed to "one" or "many". There are also monistic forms of *Vedanta*.

Vedas: The oldest and root literature of Hinduism and **brahminism** originally transmitted orally through chanting. There are four Vedas conveying religious and ritual instructions that emphasize the nature, appeasement, and enlistment of the gods. As I understand it the religion of the Vedas was primarily a priestly religion, but contained remnants of an earlier shamanism (see **shaman**).

Vichara: Various writers have interpreted this as "pondering", "philosophical discrimination", or "thinking". See **subtle objects**.

Virtuality: This designates the "realm" of virtual knowledge and related imagery arising from language alone, i.e., without dependence on immediate sensory process. This is not the same as "**imaginal**", however, since all experience actual and virtual depends upon **imagination**. See also **fancy**.

Withdrawal of the senses (*pratyahara*): The fifth limb of the **tree of yoga** in which one turns attention away from the outer world of the senses toward the inner world of feelings and mental process. It also represents turning to the practices of the **inner discipline** having attained a degree of grounding in the **outer discipline**. This does not mean, however, that practice of the outer discipline is abandoned. Each of the eight limbs supports the others. Withdrawal of the senses should not be viewed as a renunciation or rejection of the sensory world, but as a technique of self-discipline in which indifference to sensory stimulation is cultivated in favor of one-pointed concentration within.

Yantra: *Yantra* are geometric devices used for meditative concentration. They may be actual objects drawn or painted for the purpose, or internally generated visualizations. The word means "device" or "vehicle" and could apply to many yogic tools. Some *yantra* represent deities while others are intended to reflect metaphysical ideas. In *tantra* the human body is considered a *yantram* thus relating *hatha* yoga practices to concentration.

Yoga: From the Indo-European root "yuj". This is the same as the root of "yoke" and may have originally meant yoke. The implication is one of harnessing energy and keeping it on track (focused, concentrated) for the purpose of tilling mental "soil".

Yogi: One who practices yogic techniques with a high degree of mastery. The latter refers to success at removing obstacles and attenuating ignorance. The vast majority of practitioners are, in my opinion, more accurately referred to as "practitioners", or "students" of yoga.

Yogasutra of Patanjali: A collection of aphorisms written down sometime around 200 C.E. that represent the principle text of **classical yoga**. The work is more psycho-technical than philosophical.

Yogini: A female *yogi*.

Zafu: A Japanese word denoting a round, somewhat fat and firm cushion used for sitting meditation. As far as I know the *zafu* was first introduced to the West by Zen Buddhists.

Index

978-0-595-39368-8
0-595-39368-3